Laser Management of Scars

Kayvan Shokrollahi
Editor

Laser Management of Scars

Springer

Editor
Kayvan Shokrollahi
Burns and Plastic Surgery Unit
Whiston Hospital
Liverpool
UK

ISBN 978-3-030-52918-5   ISBN 978-3-030-52919-2 (eBook)
https://doi.org/10.1007/978-3-030-52919-2

This Springer imprint is published by the registered company Springer Nature Switzerland AG
The registered company address is: Gewerbestrasse 11, 6330 Cham, Switzerland

Preface

Within these pages, I have endeavoured to bring together the current state of the art of laser technology and its application to the problem of cutaneous scarring.

Scar management is a very challenging field. One of the biggest challenges is the variability of scars—ranging from aetiology, severity, distribution, skin type of the patient, comorbidities, genetics, age and changeability with time and compliance, to name but a few. This presents the dilemma that no two scars are the same, that there is no 'standard' scar in our patients, and that the numbers of scars of a certain type (when variables are matched) are low or unmatchable in most study populations. There is patient and observer subjectivity in the assessment of scars, and some of the most important aspect of scars in the eyes of patients such as whether they can be covered or not with camouflage is not an acknowledged clinical end point, nor has an outcome measure. In relation to objective outcomes, the field is in its infancy and not at a point where it is of practical use in clinical practice. Photography in the assessment of scars is extremely challenging and difficult to standardise.

Nowhere are these challenges greater than in a clinical sphere that is close to my heart, burn care—to answer the 'big questions' in this patient group, we really need a decade's worth of data possibly with a supra-national size data set. Hence, despite best efforts and research over decades, the quality of evidence 'out there' for scar interventions remains poor compared to most fields of clinical and scientific endeavour. Yet despite these challenges, clinicians and scientists continue to strive to bring to bear clinical and scientific strategies to deliver the most effective treatments for their patients.

One intervention that has gained substantial traction in scar management over the last decades is lasers. These highly sophisticated devices by their nature present a number of challenges of their own when brought to bear on scar problems, including:

- Expense.
- Significant variability of lasers even of the same general type, between laser manufacturers.
- Expertise, training and availability.
- The narrow spectrum of indications for use of any one specific type of laser; the unique defining 'single-wavelength' characteristic of lasers at the heart of their clinical utility typically limits their utility to a single-scar trait.
- The requirement for a suite of lasers to deal with the full spectrum of scar problems.
- The requirement for multiple treatments, sometimes over a prolonged period of time.
- The range of different lasers available: even the same wavelength of laser made by different manufacturers is difficult to compare, as by nature of the fact that each machine is marketed and created to be better than others, all have their own settings, nuances and special features that are not comparable between machines.

When comparing the challenges already faced in the realms of scar assessment with these additional hurdles unique to lasers, it is clear that there may be insurmountable challenges in obtaining the levels of evidence and objective outcomes we desire any time soon. There is, however, one saving grace: our patients are as invested as us in making scars better: by listening to them, gaining their feedback, and shaping our practice there remains hope for the future.

Liverpool, UK
2020

Kayvan Shokrollahi

Acknowledgements

I am most grateful to all the contributors that have helped bring this project to fruition.

Springer-Nature has been a truly professional (and patient) publisher that has worked tirelessly to get this book over the line. Many thanks to Jordan Ewing for some administrative assistance.

Special thanks to the patients who helped to disseminate knowledge through discussion of their cases.

Finally, a personal word of thanks to all authors whose work we were not able to include in the final manuscript.

Contents

Contributors

Andrea Bassi Laser Cutaneous Cosmetic and Plastic Surgery Unit, Villa Donatello Clinic, Florence, Italy

David Bodansky Department of Orthopaedic Surgery, Royal Liverpool Hospital, Liverpool, UK

Mersey Regional Burns and Plastic Surgery Unit, St Helens and Knowsley Teaching Hospitals NHS Trust, Prescot, Merseyside, UK

Paolo Bonan Laser Cutaneous Cosmetic and Plastic Surgery Unit, Villa Donatello Clinic, Florence, Italy

Ludwik K. Branski Division of Plastic Surgery, Department of Surgery, The University of Texas Medical Branch, Shriners Hospital for Children, Galveston, TX, USA

Mark Brewin Salisbury Laser Clinic, Salisbury NHS Foundation Trust, Salisbury, Wiltshire, UK

Nicola Bruscino Laser Cutaneous Cosmetic and Plastic Surgery Unit, Villa Donatello Clinic, Florence, Italy

Amanda Champlain Division of Dermatology, Loyola University Chicago, Chicago, IL, USA

Charlotte Defty Mersey Regional Centre for Burns and Plastic Surgery, Whiston Hospital, Liverpool, UK

Gerd G. Gauglitz Department of Dermatology and Allergy, Ludwig-Maximilian-University, Munich, Germany

Parneet Gill Mersey Regional Centre for Burns and Plastic Surgery, Whiston Hospital, Liverpool, UK

Charlotte Hardman Mersey Regional Centre for Burns and Plastic Surgery, Whiston Hospital, Liverpool, UK

Swati Kannan Department of Dermatology, Kaiser Southern California Permanente Medical Group, Riverside, CA, USA

Corina Lavelle The Christie NHS Foundation Trust, Manchester, UK

Jillian M. McLaughlin Division of Plastic Surgery, Department of Surgery, The University of Texas Medical Branch, Shriners Hospital for Children, Galveston, TX, USA

Adeyinka Molajo Mersey Regional Centre for Burns and Plastic Surgery, Whiston Hospital, Liverpool, UK

Lauren Moy Division of Dermatology, Loyola University Chicago, Chicago, IL, USA

Umarah Muhammad Mersey Regional Centre for Burns and Plastic Surgery, Whiston Hospital, Liverpool, UK

William B. Norbury Division of Plastic Surgery, Department of Surgery, The University of Texas Medical Branch, Shriners Hospital for Children, Galveston, TX, USA

Rei Ogawa Department of Plastic, Reconstructive and Aesthetic Surgery, Nippon Medical School, Tokyo, Japan

Youssof Oskrochi Royal Liverpool and Broadgreen University Hospitals NHS Trust, Liverpool, UK

David Ozog Department of Dermatology, Henry Ford Hospital, Detroit, MI, USA

Anne Le Pillouer-Prost Service de Dermatologie, Hôpital Privé Clairval, Marseille, France

Julian Poetschke Department of Dermatology and Allergy, Ludwig-Maximilian-University, Munich, Germany

Department of Plastic and Handsurgery, Burn Center, Klinikum St. Georg gGmbH, Leipzig, Germany

Jared L. Potts Division of Plastic Surgery, Department of Surgery, The University of Texas Medical Branch, Shriners Hospital for Children, Galveston, TX, USA

Nastaran Sargazi Mersey Regional Burns and Plastic Surgery Unit, St Helens and Knowsley Teaching Hospitals NHS Trust, Prescot, Merseyside, UK

Emiliano Schincaglia Laser Cutaneous Cosmetic and Plastic Surgery Unit, Villa Donatello Clinic, Florence, Italy

Kayvan Shokrollahi Burns and Plastic Surgery Unit, Whiston Hospital, Liverpool, UK

Yvonne Stubbington Mersey Regional Centre for Burns and Plastic Surgery, Whiston Hospital, Liverpool, UK

David Surprenant Division of Dermatology, Loyola University Chicago, Chicago, IL, USA

Joy Tao Division of Dermatology, Loyola University Chicago, Chicago, IL, USA

Luke Taylor Mersey Regional Centre for Burns and Plastic Surgery, Whiston Hospital, Liverpool, UK

Michela Troiano Laser Cutaneous Cosmetic and Plastic Surgery Unit, Villa Donatello Clinic, Florence, Italy

Rebecca Tung Florida Dermatology and Skin Cancer Centers, Winter Haven, FL, USA

Charles Weddington Department of Dermatology, University of Maryland, Baltimore, MD, USA

Dexter W. Weeks Division of Plastic Surgery, Department of Surgery, The University of Texas Medical Branch, Shriners Hospital for Children, Galveston, TX, USA

About the Author

Kayvan Shokrollahi is a Burns, Plastic and Laser Surgeon at the Mersey Regional Centre for Burns and Plastic Surgery, Merseyside, UK, and Deputy Chair of the British Burn Association. He is the editor-in-chief of the journal *Scars Burns & Healing* (SAGE) and associate editor of *Annals of Plastic Surgery* (Lippincott). He has authored and edited a number of well-respected textbooks in the field of burns and plastic surgery including *Burns* (Oxford Specialist handbook series) and *Flaps: Practical Reconstructive Surgery* (Thieme), amongst others.

Introduction to Lasers and Their Use in Scar Management

Kayvan Shokrollahi

1 Principles of Laser–Tissue Interactions

Laser light, when delivered into tissue, interacts in a number of different ways. These specific interactions depend on the tissue type, wavelength of the laser as well as the laser energy delivered into the tissues (fluence). A laser beam will continue to travel through tissue until it is absorbed, and the specific entity within the skin that absorbs that energy is known as the chromophore. Three main chromophores of therapeutic relevance reside in the skin:

- Haemoglobin (blood)
- Melanin (skin pigment)
- Water

Vascular lasers are absorbed well by haemoglobin and exert their therapeutic effects through this absorption. Hence, a vascular scar or area of telangiectasia will absorb laser energy and (for instance) result in coagulation or disruption of fine vessels.

Lasers that target melanin are useful for depilation, and in some circumstances for treatment of pigmentation.

Lasers that target water are typically ablative lasers which cause a degree of tissue destruction, acting superficially at first and penetrating deeper dependant on the power of the laser used, the pulse duration, and the method and duration of delivery. Lasers such as the CO_2 laser can be deployed either as a single beam or as various larger patterns through use of a computer pattern generator (CPG) that can not only treat larger areas in one go but also 'fractionate' the delivery of the laser energy to spare selected densities of tissue to allow for more rapid and consistent healing with reduced 'downtime' and with reduced risk.

With the appropriate selection of laser (wavelength), fluence (energy and density) and pulse duration, and other factors, selective destruction of a specific target becomes possible—termed selective photothermolysis. The depth of the skin penetration, from epidermis down to subcutaneous tissue, varies depending on the wavelength of laser light, spot size, amount of chromophore, and various other factors.

2 Scar Characteristics Commonly Amenable to Laser Therapy

- Erythema
- Dyschromia, hyperpigmentation, and hypopigmentation
- Atrophy
- Telangiectasia
- Contour
- Pliability
- Scar folliculitis
- Iatrogenic, e.g. 'post-corticosteroid', post-meshed skin grafts, and heterotopic hair.

3 Providing a Laser Scar Service

Most scars have more than one treatable problem, e.g. erythema + pigmentation + texture and patients themselves have different skin types (I to VI). These different scars in different patients require different lasers and different strategies to deal with all the variables. It is simply not possible to have a 'one-laser' approach to all scars, and indeed such a strategy can lead to poor results or itself cause complications or scarring. Therefore, a comprehensive suite of lasers is typically required including:

- Vascular lasers
- Ideally long-pulsed pulsed dye and/or Nd:YAG lasers

K. Shokrollahi (✉)
Burns and Plastic Surgery Unit, Whiston Hospital, Liverpool, UK

K. Shokrollahi (ed.), *Laser Management of Scars*, https://doi.org/10.1007/978-3-030-52919-2_1

- Depilatory lasers
- Such as Alexandrite, diode, and Nd:YAG (for type 5 or 6 skin)
- Ablative lasers
- Primarily carbon dioxide lasers, but also erbium:YAG. These should be able to deliver ablative and fractionated delivery.

Patient expectations will need to be managed appropriately, and laser will typically fit into a treatment regime encompassing multiple different modalities such as:

- Corticosteroid injections or other topical drug interventions
- Cosmetic camouflage
- Pressure garments (burns)
- Topical silicone
- Massage (physical or mechanical)
- Surgery, dermabrasion, needling

Patients with scars are ideally managed in the context of a scar MDT with multiple modalities on offer including laser and with access to counselling and mental health support.

Laser are not a panacea and there must be appropriate expectations from clinicians and patients alike. The one thing that patients want from scar treatments is the thing they cannot have: the 'removal' of their scars. A holistic approach including camouflage, ancillary treatments, and psychological input as needed are essential.

Clinicians have yet to develop the objective and patient-reported measures needed to evaluate laser treatments in the areas where it can make the most difference—for example the ability of patients to cover their scars with camouflage or makeup. Simultaneous with the development and expansion of light-based interventions for scar management, we also need to come out of the dark when it comes to the development of objective measures, subjective measures, patient-reported measures, and aspects such as camouflagability of scarring. There are huge challenges in this area because every scar and injury is different, every patient is different and has a different skin type, the anatomical location of scars are different, the mechanisms of injury and depths are different, and the co-morbidities are different. When combined with the essential requirement for many patients to have, for clinical reasons, multimodal treatments, this presents potentially insurmountable challenges in this area.

We must both recognise these challenges and strive to capture the best evidence. We must be cognisant that the world evidence in this domain is mostly based in level 4 and 5 evidence and case series.

Further Reading

Lindsay KJ, Shokrollahi K. Laser management of scars (chap. 44). In: Whitaker IS, Shokrollahi K, Dickson WA, editors. Burns (OSH surgery). Oxford: Oxford University Press; 2019. ISBN-13: 9780199699537. https://doi.org/10.1093/med/9780199699537.001.0001.

Pathophysiology of Scarring

Nastaran Sargazi, David Bodansky, and Kayvan Shokrollahi

1 Wound Healing and Scarring

When cutaneous integrity is disrupted, wound healing and the formation of scars are essential in providing a protective barrier against infection and fluid loss [1]. Wound healing is a complex process triggered by an initial insult, which progresses in a systematic manner and is categorised into three specific phases: inflammatory, proliferative and remodelling [2]. The duration of this cascade of events varies between individuals and can take many months to complete [2].

Within minutes of the initial insult, clot formation at the wound site initiates the inflammatory phase [2] by attracting inflammatory cells, in particular neutrophils, which migrate to the area of trauma [3]. Neutrophil-specific enzymes, including collagenases, are hypothesised to contribute to scar formation by resulting in areas of excessive tissue loss, thereby leaving large defects which are ultimately replaced during the remodelling phase by scar tissue [4]. Chemotactic agents also result in migration of monocytes to the region of injury which are transformed into macrophages on reaching the wound site and not only act in an inflammatory manner but also play a vital role in the proliferative phase by stimulating angiogenesis and re-epithelialisation [5].

The proliferative phase ensues over the next few days to weeks and consists of a chain of events resulting in repair of both the dermal and epidermal layers [3]. This stage involves a range of processes including angiogenesis, granulation tissue formation, deposition of collagen, re-epithelialization and retraction of the wound which ultimately results in scar formation [6]. In the process of angiogenesis, a rich network of capillaries created from surrounding healthy blood vessels are formed throughout the wound [6]. These are initially fragile and relatively permeable, resulting in a degree of tissue oedema [6].

Next, collagen deposition occurs as a result of secretion of extracellular matrix proteins by fibroblasts following their migration and proliferation in the wound [6].The resulting vascularised, pink fibrous tissue is termed granulation tissue and acts to replace the clot previously formed at the site of trauma [6]. Once adequate quantities of matrix are laid down, fibroblasts differentiate into myofibroblasts and initiate wound contraction [6]. Re-epithelialisation occurs early in this process, with keratinocytes migrating from wound edges to cover the granulation tissue and proliferating across the denuded area of skin [5], thereby differentiating into a new layer of epidermis [3]. In its final stage, the wound enters the maturation phase during which the granulation tissue undergoes remodelling by its constituent cells, thereby allowing organisation of the scar [3].

Scar formation is the normal physiological response to cutaneous trauma [7]; however, the complex interaction that occurs between the numerous cells and their inflammatory mediators during the process of healing does not necessarily result in the formation of smooth and normal skin [8]. Dysregulation, in particular stages of the healing process, results in abnormal collagen deposition, hence, leading to excessive scar formation [9], thereby resulting in a spectrum of scar types [10], of which three are particularly amenable to laser treatment: atrophic scars, hypertrophic scars and keloids [11].

1.1 Hypertrophic Scars

Hypertrophic scars occur following an exaggerated proliferative response to wound healing [12], which results in excess collagen deposition [13]that by definition characteristically remain within the boundaries of the original wound [12]. Clinically, they appear as raised, itchy, erythematous, nodular lesions which are frequently found in areas of thicker skin [12]. They are normally present within 1 month of the initial

N. Sargazi · D. Bodansky
Mersey Regional Burns and Plastic Surgery Unit, St Helens and Knowsley Teaching Hospitals NHS Trust, Prescot, Merseyside, UK

K. Shokrollahi (✉)
Burns and Plastic Surgery Unit, Whiston Hospital, Liverpool, UK

K. Shokrollahi (ed.), *Laser Management of Scars*, https://doi.org/10.1007/978-3-030-52919-2_2

injury, regress with time and are categorised into two types: linear and widespread [13].

The linear subtype is a rope-like lesion which usually occurs following direct trauma or surgery whilst the widespread subtype is found following burns, extensive cutaneous trauma or infection [13]. Histologically, hypertrophic scars consist of disorganised arrangement of collagen assembled in a whorl-like pattern instead of the usual parallel orientation found in normal skin, giving it its characteristic raised appearance [12].Current literature shows a great range in the incidence of hypertrophic scars, with estimated rates of 30–91% following burns and 40–94% following surgery [14]. This large variation in rates has been attributed to inconsistencies in its correct identification [14].

1.2 Keloid Scars

In contrast to hypertrophic scars, keloid scars are characteristically more extensive and by definition extend beyond the margins of the wound, therefore invade normal adjacent skin [15]. Like hypertrophic scars, they are benign hyperproliferative growths developing from dense fibrous tissue following abnormal wound healing [12]. Histologically, they consist of nodules of thickened collagen bundles with relatively few fibroblasts [16], which pathognomonically invade the normal dermal layer of skin, thereby resulting in a subcutaneous mass [17]. Clinically, this results in a characteristic raised, pruritic and often painful scar which extends beyond the wound margins [18]. They can be differentiated into minor or major keloids, with the latter being larger (>0.5 cm) and more pronounced [18]. Despite their unclear aetiology, keloids tend to occur within 12 months of localised trauma, which can be in the form of surgery, tattoos, lacerations, bites, vaccinations or blunt trauma [19] and generally fail to regress with time [16].

Both hypertrophic scars and keloids form in all races; however, there is a greater predisposition in individuals with darker skin and those with greater pigment production [19]. In addition, other variables including genetic factors, hormonal levels and age play a role in the formation of such lesion [14], with most keloids occurring between the age of 10 and 30 years [19]. Furthermore, both these scars have a propensity to develop in areas exhibiting high tension [20] and slow wound healing in addition to movement- and pressure-dependent areas [13], with keloids commonly found over the earlobes, upper arm, upper back and the anterior chest, in particular the pre-sternal area [16].

The clinical distinction between keloid and hypertrophic scars is of great importance in establishing the correct management plan, in particular when deciding on the mode of laser management [16]. In general, whilst both scars tend to result from a similar pathological process, the main distinguishing features are the extension of the scar beyond the wound margin and failure to regress over time which is seen with keloids alone [20]. Further distinguishing features are described in more detail in Table 1.

Table 1 Features of hypertrophic vs. keloid scars [7]

	Keloids	Hypertrophic scars
Incidence	Rare	Common
Growth beyond wound edges	Yes	No
Pruritic	Yes	Mildly
Painful	Yes	Rarely
Predominant sites	Earlobes Anterior chest Upper arm Upper shoulder Upper back Posterior neck Knees	Extensor surface of joints Skin creases
Associated contractures	Yes	No
Stage of development	≥3 months after initial scar	Within 1 month of initial scar
Genetic predisposition	Strong link	Less genetic predisposition
Regression	No regression	Regresses with time
Recurrence rates post excision	High	Low

1.3 Atrophic Scars

Atrophic scars are a well-documented complication of acne [21], resulting from inflammatory changes which lead to dermal fat and collagen loss [22]. Clinically, they are present as broad, oval-like dermal depressions, which classically peaks in incidence during late teens to early adulthood [23]. Histologically, the loss of dermal collagen and fat results in downward displacement of the epidermis, thereby resulting in these characteristic lesions [23].These generally tend to worsen with time due to increased laxity of the skin with age [22].

In addition to the clinical impact of the scars described above, such defects can be disfiguring and hence lead to significant cosmetic concerns by patients, therefore result in considerable emotional, physical and psychological distress [10]. Consequently, a great deal of research has been undertaken within this field in order to minimise the impact of such lesions and avoid further progression [10]. Whilst a range of medical and topical agents are available for the management of such scars, this book focuses on the various laser modalities available and their place within the overall scar management pathway.

References

1. Van der Veer WM, Bloemen MCT, Ulrich MMW, Molema G, van PPM Z, Middelkoop E, et al. Potential cellular and molecular causes of hypertrophic scar formation. Burns. 2009;35(1):15–29.
2. Butler PD, Longaker MT, Yang GP. Current progress in keloid research and treatment. J Am Coll Surg. 2008;206(4):731–41.
3. Rhett JM, Ghatnekar GS, Palatinus JA, Q'Quinn M, Yost MJ, Gourdie RG. Novel therapies for scar reduction and regenerative healing of skin wounds. Trends Biotechnol. 2008;26:173–80.
4. Reish RG, Eriksson E. Scar treatments: preclinical and clinical studies. J Coll Surg. 2008;206:719–30.
5. Waibel JS, Rudnick A. Current trends and future considerations in scar treatment. Semin Cutan Med Surg J. 2015;34:13–6.
6. Young A, McNaught C. The physiology of wound healing. Surgery. 2011;29:10.
7. Arno AI, Gauglitz GG, Barret JP, Jeschke MG. Up-to-date approach to manage keloids and hypertrophic scars: a useful guide. Burns. 2014;40:1255–66.
8. Alster TS, West TB. Treatment of scars: a review. Ann Plast Surg. 1997;39:418–32.
9. Enoch S, Leaper DJ. Basic science of wound healing. Surgery. 2008;26:31–7.
10. Monstrey S, Middelkoop E, Vranckx JJ, Bassetto F, Ziegler UE, Meaume S, Téot L. Updated scar management practical guidelines: non-invasive and invasive measures. J Plast Reconstruct Aesthet Surg. 2014;67:1017–25.
11. Elsaie ML, Choudhary S, McLeod M, Nouri K. Scars. Curr Prob Dermatol. 2011;42:131–9.
12. Zurada JM, Kriegel D, Davis IC. Topical treatments for hypertrophic scars. J Am Acad Dermatol. 2006;55:1024–31.
13. Khatri KA, Mahoney DL, McCartney MJ. Laser scar revision: a review. J Cosmet Laser Ther. 2011;13:54–62.
14. Bloemen MC, van der Veer WM, Ulrich MM, van Zuijlen PP, Niessen FB, Middelkoop E. Prevention and curative management of hypertrophic scar formation. Burns. 2009;35:463–75.
15. Robles DT, Berg D. Abnormal wound healing: keloids. Clin Dermatol. 2007;25:26–32.
16. Lee JY, Yang CC, Chao SC, Wong TW. Histopathological differential diagnosis of keloid and hypertrophic Scar. Am J Dermatopathol. 2004;26:379–84.
17. Durani P, Bayat A. Levels of evidence for the treatment of keloid disease. J Plast Reconstruct Aesthet Surg. 2008;61:4–17.
18. Murray JC, Pollack SV, Pinnell SR. Keloids: a review. J Am Acad Dermatol. 1984;4:4.
19. Murray JC. Keloids and hypertrophic scars. Clin Dermatol. 1994;12:27–37.
20. Mafong EA, Ashinoff R. Treatment of hypertrophic scars and keloids: a review. Aesthet Surg J. 2000;20:2.
21. Woo SH, Park JH, Kye YC. Resurfacing of different types of facial acne scar with short-pulsed, variable-pulsed, and dual-mode Er:YAG laser. Dermatol Surg. 2004;30:488–93.
22. O'Daniel TG. Multimodal management of atrophic acne scarring in the aging face. Aesthetic Plast Surg. 2011;35:1143–50.
23. Jordan R, Cummins C, Buris A. Laser resurfacing of the skin for the improvement of facial acne scarring: a systematic review of the evidence. Br J Dermatol. 2000;142:413–23.

Decision-Making for Safe and Effective Laser Treatment: The Laser Test Patch

Kayvan Shokrollahi and Charlotte Defty

1 Introduction

Laser test patching is a fundamental step in performing a laser treatment and its importance should not be overlooked. It is a frequent key in achieving the optimal result whilst avoiding complications. A test patch is carried out to help select the most effective, safe treatment as smoothly as possible, whilst avoiding overtreating and the resultant adverse effects. Patient satisfaction with the treatment process and outcome is paramount and this is neither accomplished by undertreating patients and having no side effects nor by successfully treating the presenting complaint but leaving unnecessary scarring, pigment alteration and other problems. Test patching also demonstrates that steps were taken to avoid complications and can play an important role in supporting the clinician's practice if adverse effects were to arise. There are however circumstances when a test patch is neither practical nor beneficial.

2 General Principles of Performing a Test Patch [1]

A test patch should be performed in most laser treatments to help select the most effective laser settings for the condition and site being treated according to Shokrollahi's principles [1]. The aim of test patching is to define parameters which are maximally effective, safe and have minimal adverse effects, following which full treatments can be performed with confidence. Decisions regarding the parameters for the test patch are based on the underlying condition, the skin type of the patient, the anatomical site and the laser being used [2]. A range of parameters usually within the manufacturer's recommendations should be tried. Straying beyond manufacturers parameters is not a problem in itself and can often be required to get the desired clinical end points. Appropriate test patching and meticulous informed consent will therefore underpin advanced laser practitioners as they push the equipment to the limits whilst maximising safety and effectiveness and whilst understanding that a good result for one patient may be disappointing to another due to the subjectivity of outcomes in this field—again underscoring the importance of the test patch.

Different test patches are required for different anatomical areas, as skin sensitivity, quality and thickness varies considerably. This factor, as well as attempting to conceal the test patch in case of problems, must be considered when choosing the site. For example, the pre-auricular area provides a comparable skin type to the rest of the face when planning facial resurfacing. Different test patches should be performed to represent the different anatomical areas which are to be treated, and if the effectiveness is not optimal, the parameters can be increased in small steps. The environment for the test patching such as the pre- or post-cooling regime should be the same as that for the full treatment, if the laser parameters chosen can be relied upon. Repeating the test patching must also be considered after the laser has been calibrated.

Aside from assessing the suitable parameters for the full treatment, a test patch also has the added advantage of demonstrating to the patient a sample of what is to be expected from the procedure and the recovery period. By doing this, the patient has a much better understanding of the treatment to which they are consenting.

There are however situations when a test patch may not be useful or practical. These include some ablative procedures such as when using a laser to incise tissue or ablate a scar. It is also not practical when the treatment is so small that the test patch is the treatment. If the laser practitioner feels that a test patch is not appropriate, they need to be able to justify this decision and, if felt necessary, discuss this with the patient.

K. Shokrollahi (✉)
Burns and Plastic Surgery Unit, Whiston Hospital, Liverpool, UK

C. Defty
Mersey Regional Centre for Burns and Plastic Surgery, Whiston Hospital, Liverpool, UK

K. Shokrollahi (ed.), *Laser Management of Scars*, https://doi.org/10.1007/978-3-030-52919-2_3

3 Safety and Effectiveness of Test Patching in Relation to Treating Scars

Lasers can be used to treat a range of different unwanted characteristics of scars, and test patching may or may not be required depending on the type of scar and the modality of treatment. If a scar is a source of distress in the eyes of the patient, leading to their desire for treatment to improve the appearance, the risk of any adverse effects and worsening of the scar must be minimised and discussed with the patient. The focus of the laser treatment may be on the contour or lumpiness of the scar, the thickened quality as in burn scarring, the effects on the surrounding tissue, a general hyperaemia or specific prominent vessels within the scar among other features. Any treatment has a measurable risk of worsening the appearance and this must be weighed carefully against the likely benefits. ‘Surgical’ style laser treatments for scars may not warrant rigorous test patching, whereas non-ablative or ablative treatments such as vascular or resurfacing treatments will variably be more suited. For multiple scars, ‘trial of laser’ may be a more appropriate strategy where laser treatment is provided to one of the smallest of a range of scars to gauge the improvement and outcome and risk of adverse effects.

In most cases of treating unwanted vascular characteristics, a test patch should be performed on the least conspicuous area of the scar using the general principles described above. The exception to this is when the test patch is the full treatment. In the case of ablative procedures for raised scars or associated ridges or lumps, the advantages and disadvantages of performing a test patch must be evaluated. Factors to consider include the size of the scar, whether general, local or topical anaesthetic are required for the full treatment, the recovery process and any downtime for the patient. In very large areas, it may be unwise to treat the whole area without a test patch, not only because of potential undesired adverse effects but because of minimal or no improvement. There may be a significant downtime from this type of treatment and if little benefit results, this would be dissatisfactory for the patient. The risk of this could be minimised by performing a test patch with little or no downtime. Following a test patch in this case, the patient is able to make an informed decision as to whether to proceed with a treatment of the full area.

In some larger full treatments, when a general anaesthetic may be required, knowledge of the effective safe parameters with which to proceed as defined by a test patch under local anaesthetic may reduce unnecessary general anaesthetic procedures. An example of this would be in performing a test patch on part of a large burn scar plaque. Following this, treatment of the larger area can proceed under general anaesthetic with the reassurance that there would likely be a positive outcome.

In the case of small scars such as a ridge on the edge of a full thickness skin graft, performing a test patch and then the full treatment would double the procedures required and recovery and downtime for the patient for little or no benefit.

4 Conclusion

Test patching is an important step in the majority of laser treatments. It is not simply a tick-box exercise, and the reasons for doing or not doing it should be assessed on an individual basis. When it is appropriate, it is important to consider the site and parameters which should be tested in order to gain maximum benefit from the test patch and subsequent treatment. When it is not undertaken, this must be justified and explained to the patient prior to proceeding with the full treatment.

References

1. Shokrollahi K. The laser test patch: principles and philosophy to maximise efficacy and reduce complications and scarring from laser treatments. Ann Plast Surg. 2016;77(4):373–5. https://doi.org/10.1097/SAP.0000000000000894.
2. Shokrollahi K, Raymond E, Murison MS. Lasers: principles and surgical applications. J Surg. 2004;2:28–34.

Laser Strategies for Complex Scars: Experience from Establishing a Supra-Regional Laser Service for Burns and Complex Scarring

Kayvan Shokrollahi, Luke Taylor, and Parneet Gill

Abbreviations

ACO_2	Abblative carbdon dixoide laser
FCO_2	Fractionated carbdon dixoide laser
Hz	Hertz
J	Joules
PDL	Pulsed dye laser
QS	Q-switched
Rx	Treatment
UK	United Kingdom

1 Introduction

Scarring as a result of burns, trauma, or surgery affects approximately 100 million people each year across the developed world [1]. Although scars are a normal physiological response to cutaneous injury, depending on their features, they can have a widely varied impact on a patient's physical and psychological health [2, 3]. Excessive scar formation is an undesirable process of healing that occurs through uncontrolled reparative mechanisms, often leading to erythema, altered pigmentation, hypertrophic and keloid scaring, altered skin texture, pain, and functional deficits [4]. Management of the arising physical and psychosocial conditions associated with scars and burns is therefore of utmost importance, often requiring a multimodal approach [3].

The use of laser treatment in medical practice is still in its early phases, though there is increasing evidence for its benefit in the management of both burns and scars. In 2018, the UK National Burn Care Standards for the first time specified that access to laser treatments should be available for burns survivors at least within an individual burns network (NHS England operational delivery networks for burns) [5]—acknowledging the increasing evidence of benefit of laser modalities to help patients with a range of scar-related problems.

Laser light, when delivered to tissue, interacts in a number of different ways. These specific interactions depend on the tissue type, wavelength of the laser as well as the laser fluence and pulse duration [6]. A laser beam will continue to travel through tissue until it is absorbed. The laser beam will only be absorbed at the level that it no longer passes through tissue, at which point heat energy is produced causing thermal damage to the tissue [7]. It is this principle of selective absorption that makes the laser treatment of scars and burns so effective. By choosing different wavelengths of light, it is possible to target specific components of tissue and leave the surrounding structures relatively unaffected [8].With the appropriate selection of laser wavelength, fluence, density and pulse duration, selective destruction of a specific target becomes possible—termed selective photothermolysis [8]. The depth of skin penetration, from epidermis down to subcutaneous tissue, varies depending on the wavelength of laser light, with different wavelengths being absorbed by different structures. Each structure in the skin tissue will absorb a particular wavelength of laser light depending on its characteristics, allowing for deeper or more superficial penetration of laser [9].

This chapter seeks to provide a snapshot of the type of patients with scar problems that may present to a regional service with a range of complex problems and some of the laser strategies that can be deployed in their treatment.

2 Treatment Population

A snapshot of caseload of the senior author demonstrated 159 patients underwent laser treatment for the management of scars at the Mersey Regional Laser Unit, Department of

K. Shokrollahi (✉)
Burns and Plastic Surgery Unit, Whiston Hospital, Liverpool, UK

L. Taylor · P. Gill
Mersey Regional Centre for Burns and Plastic Surgery, Whiston Hospital, Liverpool, UK

K. Shokrollahi (ed.), *Laser Management of Scars*, https://doi.org/10.1007/978-3-030-52919-2_4

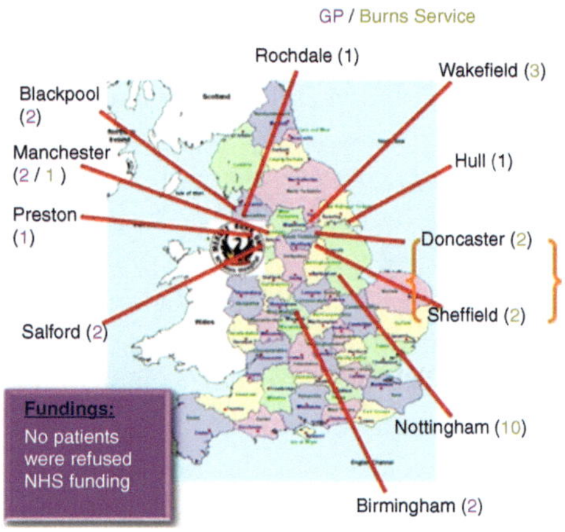

Fig. 1 Supra-regional referral patterns 2014–2016. Referrals have increased since this initial cohort of patients

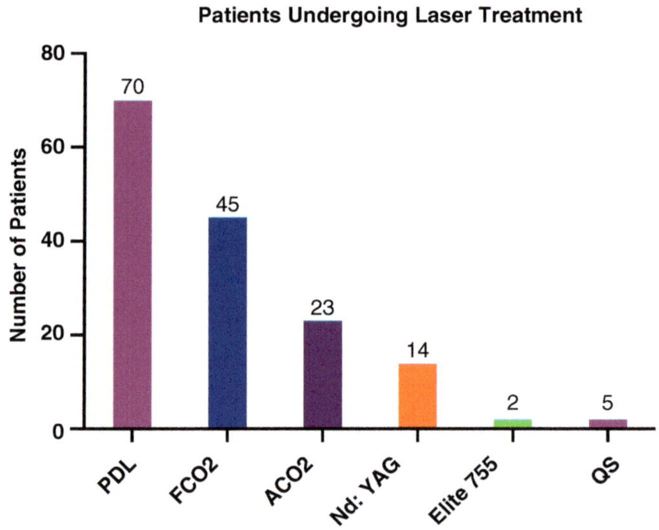

Fig. 2 Bar chart showing the number of patients undergoing treatment with each laser type of varying mediums and frequency. *PDL* pulsed dye laser, *FCO_2* fractional CO_2 laser, *ACO_2* ablative CO_2 laser, *Elite 755* alexandrite long-pulsed laser, *QS* Q-switched Nd:YAG or KTP laser

Table 1 Showing the indications for patient referral and the treatment received for each

Indications for referral	Mainstay of treatments offered
Hair (e.g. in skin grafts; folliculitis)	Injectable chemotherapy
Range of motion	Ablative CO_2 laser
Pigmentation and erythema	Fractional CO_2 laser
Contour	Pulsed dye laser
Keloid scarring	Alexandrite and Nd: YAG lasers
Special (e.g. microstomia)	Surgery

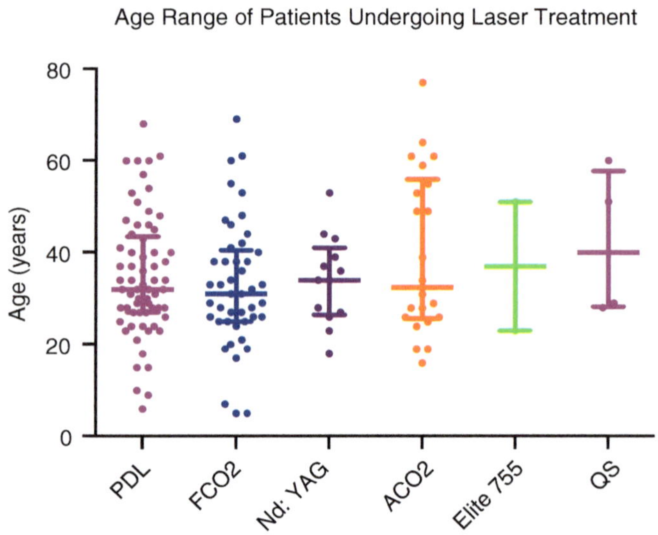

Fig. 3 Scatter plot showing the age range of patients undergoing treatment with each laser type. Error bars show median age and the upper and lower interquartile ranges

Burns and Plastic Surgery, Whiston Hospital from 2012 to 2018. During this time, the service received a significant portion of referrals from outside the region especially for treatment of burns scars, with referrals from three of the four national burn networks (Fig. 1) with indications for referral outlined in Table 1. As the availability of laser treatment has become more viable, and favourable results demonstrated clinically to referring clinicians and patients themselves, so the referrals have increased and continue to rise.

These patients have received treatment using several different lasers depending on their clinical presentation, including the pulsed dye laser (PDL), fractionated CO_2 laser (FCO_2), ablative CO_2 laser (ACO_2), elite Nd: YAG1064 laser, alexandrite laser and the Q-switched 1064 and 532 lasers. A breakdown of the number of patients receiving treatment with each laser can be seen in Fig. 2. The median age for all patients treated was 32, with an interquartile range of 26–44, and the female-to-male ratio was 104:55. Figure 3 shows a scatter plot of the age range for patients separated into treatment by each individual laser. Patients also required a varying number of treatments to reach the desired outcome, a breakdown of number of treatments required for each laser is shown in Fig. 4. A full breakdown of patient demographics for each type of laser treatment can be seen in Table 2.

3 The Laser Test Patch

All patients, except those receiving treatment with the ablative CO_2 laser, underwent test patching prior to their treatment. Laser test patches are a crucial part of providing the highest quality of treatment and the best possible outcomes for the patient [10]. This allows for selection of the most appropriate and effective laser parameters for each individual patient, within the limits of each individual laser whilst avoiding complications such as hypopigmentation, hyperpigmentation, burns, blistering, and further scarring. The most effective parameters of each laser for use in the treatment of possible scars are outlined under 'Indications for Treatment'. Readers are directed to the specific chapters on laser test patching and complications in this book.

4 Indications for Treatment

Due to the absorption spectra of laser light, there are several applications for treatment depending on the clinical need. Typical indications for laser treatment of scars include: pigmentation, erythema/telangiectasia, hypertrophic scarring, acne scarring, ectopic hair/scar folliculitis, and keloid scars. Lasers are used either individually or in combination, in order to provide the best treatment option for the patient depending their clinical presentation and desired outcome. Patients such as those with keloid scars inevitably have additional modality treatments such as intralesional corticosteroid therapy that have been variably effective prior to referral for laser treatment.

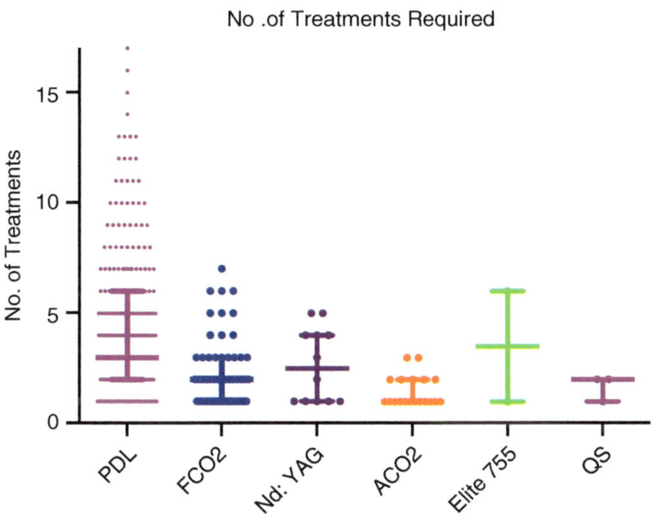

Fig. 4 Scatter plot showing the number of treatments that each patient required for each laser type to reach the desired outcome of treatment. Error bars show the median number of treatments and upper and lower interquartile ranges

5 Pigmentation

Carbon dioxide (CO_2) and Q-switched lasers provide the best treatment for areas of altered pigmentation. The CO_2 laser is an ablative laser targeting water as the chromophore that can deliver high energy precisely in short pulses either as a single beam or as a pre-selected pattern using a computer pattern generator (CPG) handpiece. As the wavelength of the CO_2 laser is readily absorbed by water, it will not penetrate deep into the tissue unless the energy levels increase, thus providing the ability for very precise tissue depth targeting depending on the clinical problem; its advantage over the main alternative ablative laser, the erbium:YAG laser, is its ability to penetrate as deep as required and its superior haemostatic properties which mean that depth penetration is unhindered by bleeding tissues which is a limitation of the erbium:YAG.

CO_2 lasers are ideal for tissue removal whilst maintaining a bloodless field as well as resurfacing of the skin to a predetermined depth and via a fractionated delivery. This makes the ablative CO_2 laser a versatile and key component in any laser scar practice, and it has the ability to treat problems related to scar contour and pigmentation in particular [11, 12].

For similar reasons, the Q-switched lasers such as Nd:YAG and frequency-doubled Nd:YAG (KTP) lasers are most commonly used in tattoo removal, and specifically target pigmentation on which they act via a photo-mechanical effect to disrupt and fragment pigmentation and promote absorption by the host immune system—in particular phagocytosis by

Table 2 Demographics of all patients undergoing laser treatment for the management of scars by the senior author

Laser	No. of patients	Median age (IQR)	F/M	Median no. of Rxs per session (IQR)	Median no. of sessions per patient (IQR)	Burn/scar
PDL	70	32 (27–43)	43/27	3 (1–4.5)	3 (2–7)	19/51
FCO_2	45	31 (25–40)	36/9	1 (1–2)	2 (2–3)	23/22
ACO_2	23	32.5 (26–54.5)	12/11	1 (1–1.75)	1 (1–2)	6/17
Nd: YAG	14	34 (27–39)	9/5	1 (1–4)	1 (1–1.75)	2/12
Alexandrite	2	37 (30–44)	0/2	3.5 (2.25–4.75)	1	1/1
QS Nd:YAG or KTP	5	40 (28.3–53.3)	4/1	1 (1–1.25)	1	3/2
Total	159	32 (26–44)	104/55	3 (1–5)	4 (2–7)	54/105

Median values and interquartile ranges are shown
PDL pulsed dye laser, *FCO_2* fractional CO_2 laser, *ACO_2* ablative CO_2 laser

macrophages [13]. These are non-ablative lasers, but due to their photo-mechanical effects are the most likely of all the non-ablative lasers to cause a degree of epidermal loss at anything other than low energies, and this should be factored into the treatment, consent, and aftercare process. Q-switched lasers have very small pulse durations (nanoseconds) and deploy considerable energy in a very short duration resulting in a palpable and audible reaction dependent on the degree of pigmentation and the amount of absorption. Newer picosecond lasers are available and these show promise for the future.

Often, there is benefit in test patching both the ablative and fractional CO_2 laser, plus non-ablative Q-switched lasers to ascertain the best response of the treatment area prior to a definitive treatment plan. The starting point for test patching pigmentation treatments in our patient group has typically been the QS Nd:YAG and/or KTP laser (at a wavelength of either 1064 or 532 nm), with a spot size of 3 mm and at an incremental fluence starting at 3.5 J/cm^2 increasing to -12.5 J/cm^2. Similarly, the ablative carbon dioxide laser is used at incremental energy levels in pulsed mode using a spot size of between 1 and 3 mm and fractional laser at high densities (for hyperpigmentation treatments) and medium energy settings on relatively small initial treatment areas. All these treatments and initial test patch parameters need to be tailored to the Fitzpatrick skin type of patients.

5.1 **Clinical Examples** (Figs. 5, 6, and 7)

5.2 Summary (Pigmentation)

Test patching with ablative lasers (Carbon dioxide, erbium:YAG) in both ablative and fractional modes, and Q-switched lasers is the best starting point for treatment of scar pigmentation using a range of suitable preliminary parameters. The skin type of the patient and underlying pathology is important to ascertain to develop a tailor-made treatment plan for each patient based on underlying anatomical, pathophysiological, and laser physics principles.

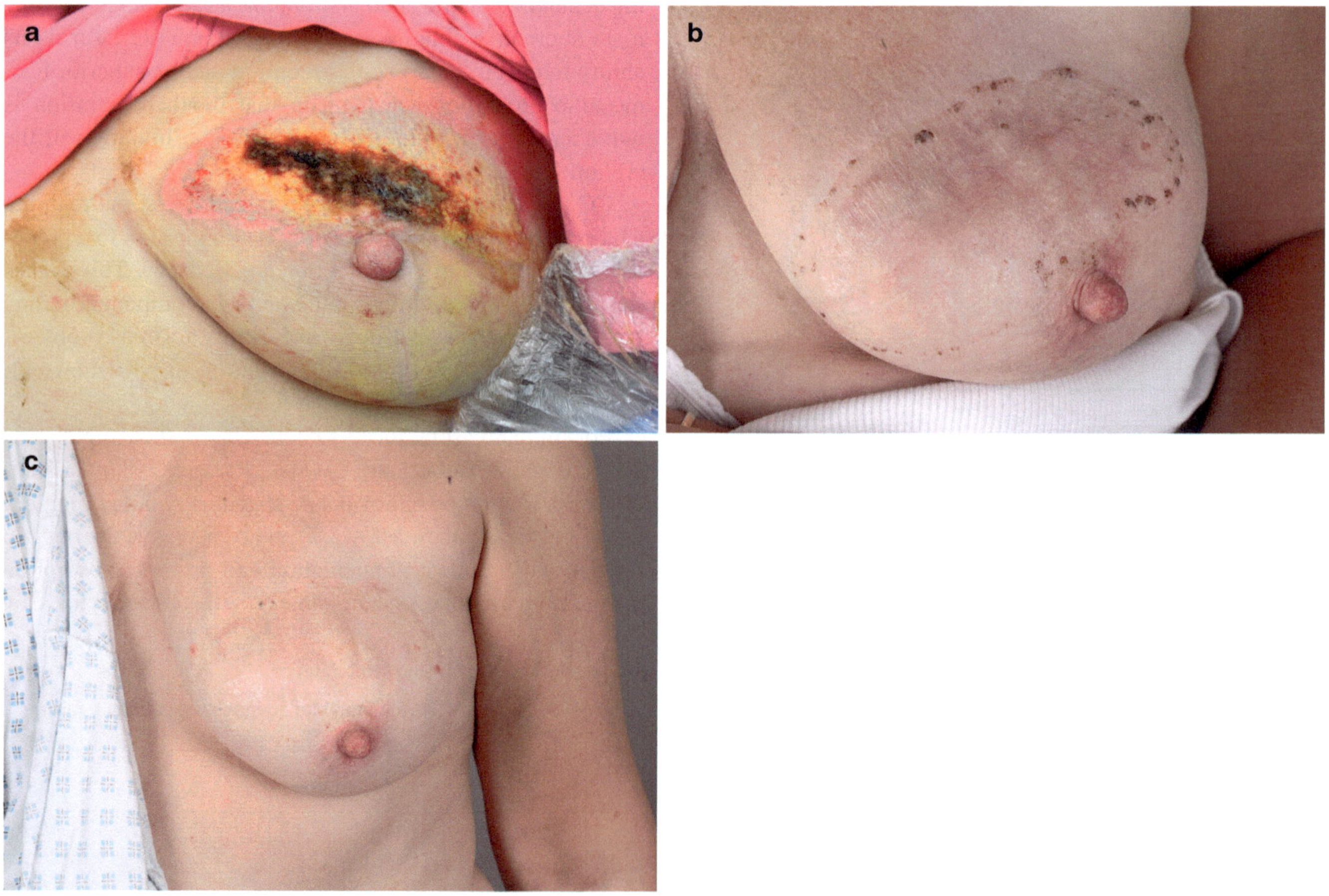

Fig. 5 (**a**) Severe deep abrasion injury after road traffic accident. (**b**) Residual pigmentation after healed. (**c**) After test patching with Q-switched and CO_2 lasers, it became apparent that the pigmentation was caused by embedded micro-shrapnel and that carbon dioxide laser was the required modality to precisely extract the shrapnel with almost complete clearance to the satisfaction of the patient

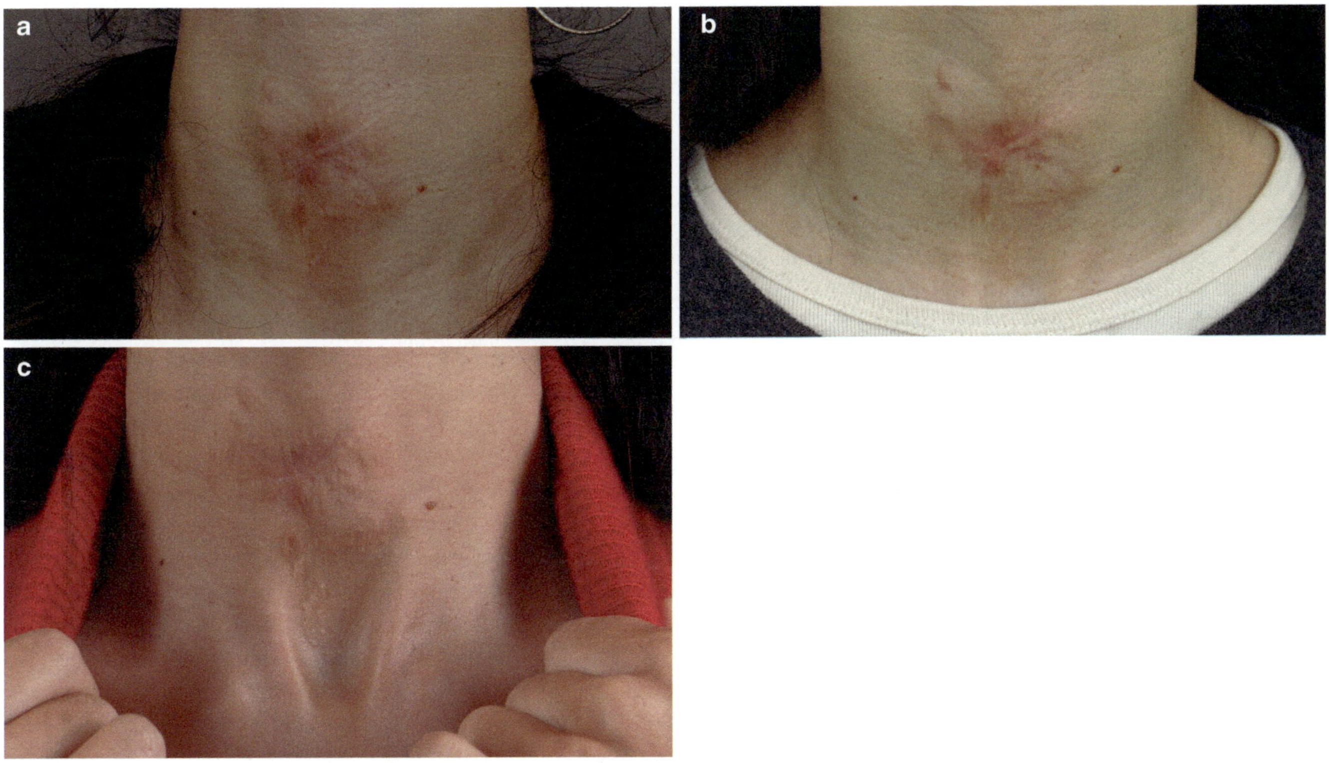

Fig. 6 (**a**) Traumatic scarring to the neck with pigmentation and contour abnormality that is difficult to disguise with camouflage. (**b**) After one sessions of carbon dioxide fractional laser resurfacing with medium energy and density settings. (**c**) After two sessions of carbon dioxide fractional laser resurfacing with medium energy and density settings, a considerable improvement was gained to the satisfaction of the patient which was compounded by the ability to cover this scar better with cosmetic camouflage

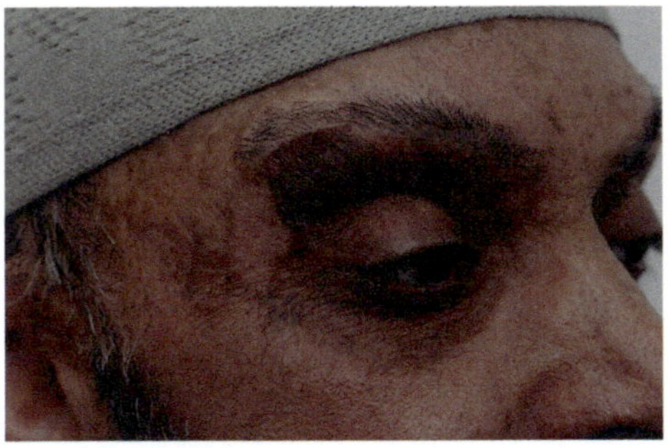

Fig. 7 Facial and periocular post-burn hyperpigmentation in a patient with Fitzpatrick type 4 skin. Pigmentary problems in dark skin types are among the most challenging problems to treat with lasers, complicated further by proximity to the eyes and the ability to only use relatively low energies. Multiple sessions of test patching may be required focussing on effective therapeutic benefit versus potential for post-inflammatory hyperpigmentation and hypopigmentation. In this case, only a very modest improvement was seen in the hyperpigmentation in some areas after test patching with Q-switched and CO_2 lasers and an initial course of treatment. Treatment was subsequently discontinued due to lack of significant benefit and long distance travel for the patient. One must always balance the potential and actual improvements achieved with the inconveniences to patients in terms of the number of treatment sessions and practicality. If the potential for improvement is limited after test patching and a number of sessions, then re-appraisal of the benefit of laser treatment should be made

Hyperpigmentation remains one of the most challenging aspects of scars to treat and requires ancillary measures including sun avoidance, high factor sun screen and may require the addition of topical bleaching agents such as hydroquinone. It remains a problem for which there is no guaranteed successful treatment, and lasers are one of a number of potential modalities that may be brought to bear on this problem. The potential for lasers to worsen the problem is an important consideration and should be factored in at all stages of consultation, test patching and consent.

6 Scar Erythema and Telangiectasia

Perhaps, the most common group of patients overall are those with vascular effects of scarring, those being erythema, hypertrophy, and telangiectasia. Vascular lasers such as the pulsed dye laser (PDL), at wavelength 595 nm, or a long-pulsed Nd: YAG laser, wavelength 1064 nm, have the best evidence base for the treatment of scars, particularly hypertrophic scars [14, 15]. Vascular lasers target the oxyhaemoglobin in the blood vessels causing thermal injury to the vessel upon light absorption [14]. It is thought that the vascular effects that reduce the erythema within scars are also the mechanisms through which other aspects of hypertrophic scarring are improved.

In our group of patients, 71 patients in the initial dataset (19 burns and 52 other scars) underwent treatment with the PDL, with a total of 352 overall treatment sessions; 14 patients underwent treatment with the long-pulsed Nd: YAG (Elite 1064) with 24 overall treatment sessions (2 burns and 12 other scars). For the PDL, the pulse duration ranged from 0.5 to 2 ms; however, in 87% of treatments, the density was set to 0.5. Spot size was consistent at either 10 or 12 mm. Fluence of the laser varied from 4 to 14 J/cm^2. All cases were undertaken without the need for any type of anaesthesia.

Whilst the longest track record for treatment of such scars is with the pulsed dye laser, significant work has been done that suggests the long-pulsed Nd:YAG laser is equally effective [16, 17], and the laser physics would suggest that deeper or purple scars would be especially suited to Nd:YAG laser treatment due to its greater depth of penetration. Due to less absorption in the epidermis, Nd:YAG is a safer laser to use for erythema in skin type 4 or greater (as is the case with laser depilation), although very little has been written on this subject matter.

Test patching with the chosen vascular laser or lasers is followed by regular sessions of a minimum of six sessions of laser for any meaningful impact to be achieved. There is no good evidence in the literature for the intervals for vascular laser treatment for scarring. Due to the extent of the problem, and in many cases extensive scarring over a wide distribution of the skin surface such as in patients with scars, it may be that treatment sessions as regular as weekly treatments are indicated to cover the often-extensive areas required and to achieve meaningful results. Survivors of major burns are likely to require multiple treatment sessions over a period of sometimes more than a year. It is unlikely that a treatment every few months for patients with extensive burn scars will achieve good results over an acceptable time frame and treatment every few weeks may be needed. In my experience, weekly treatments for severe scarring can lead to noticeable early improvements. One word of caution with a more frequent treatment regime or very large numbers of treatments is the use of the pulsed dye laser using 'purpuric' treatments typically seen with pulse durations of 0.5–2.0 ms—these can cause mild pigmentation (from likely hemosiderin deposition). It is recommended that alternating treatments with Nd:YAG laser or increasing pulse durations from 6 ms to beyond or reducing fluence to sub-purpuric settings to mitigate this problem.

There is also controversy as to when to start treatment in the course of the scarring process, but most opinions are converging on 'the sooner the better' (Figs. 8 and 9).

Pulsed dye laser tends to cause temporary skin hyperaemic changes (Fig. 10) when used at high energies with low pulse durations ('purpuric settings') which typically last for a few days and patients should be aware of this especially for facial treatments:

Scar telangiectasia is often seen either as a result of the scar or injury or as a result of treatment such as from intralesional corticosteroids. Vascular laser treatment is the main-

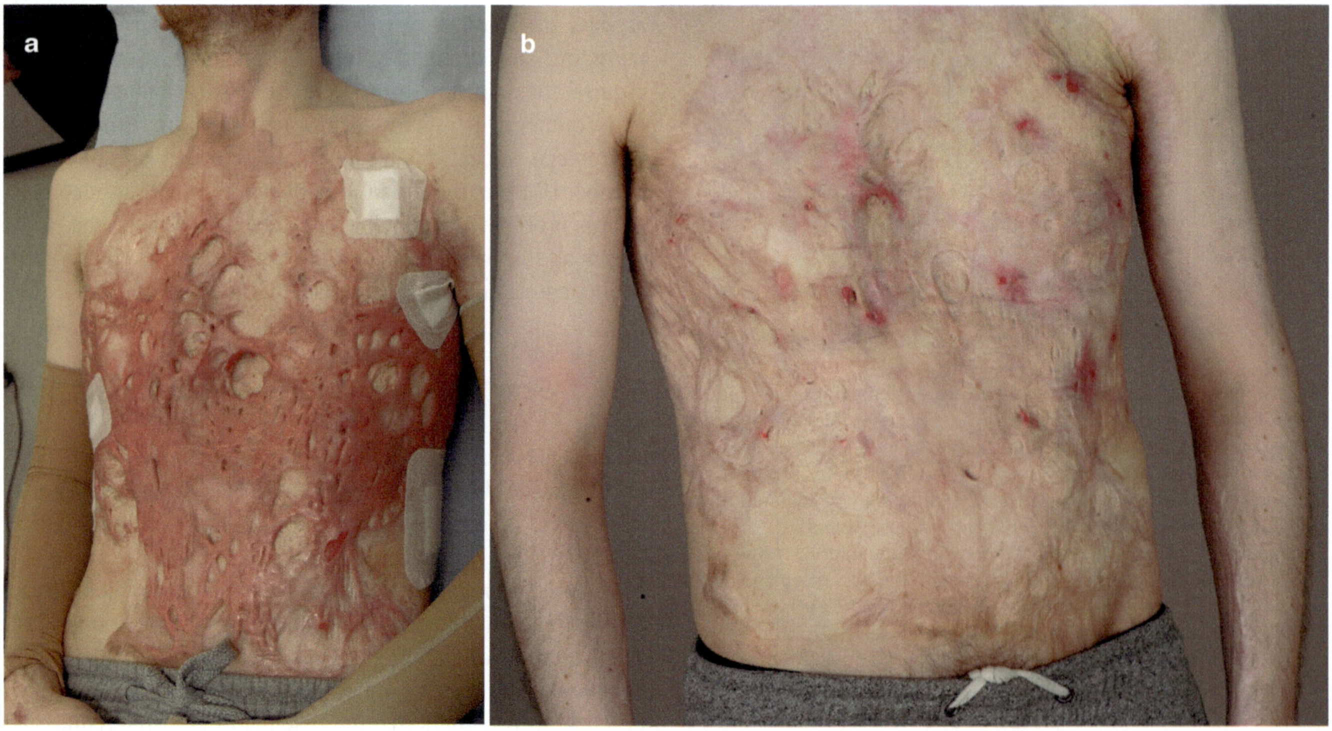

Fig. 8 (**a**) Extensive hypertrophic burn scars prior to ten sessions of pulsed dye laser treatment. (**b**) Extensive hypertrophic burn scars after ten sessions of pulsed dye laser treatment (Spot size 12, fluence 6–6.5 mJ/cm^2, pulse duration 0.5 or 2 ms)

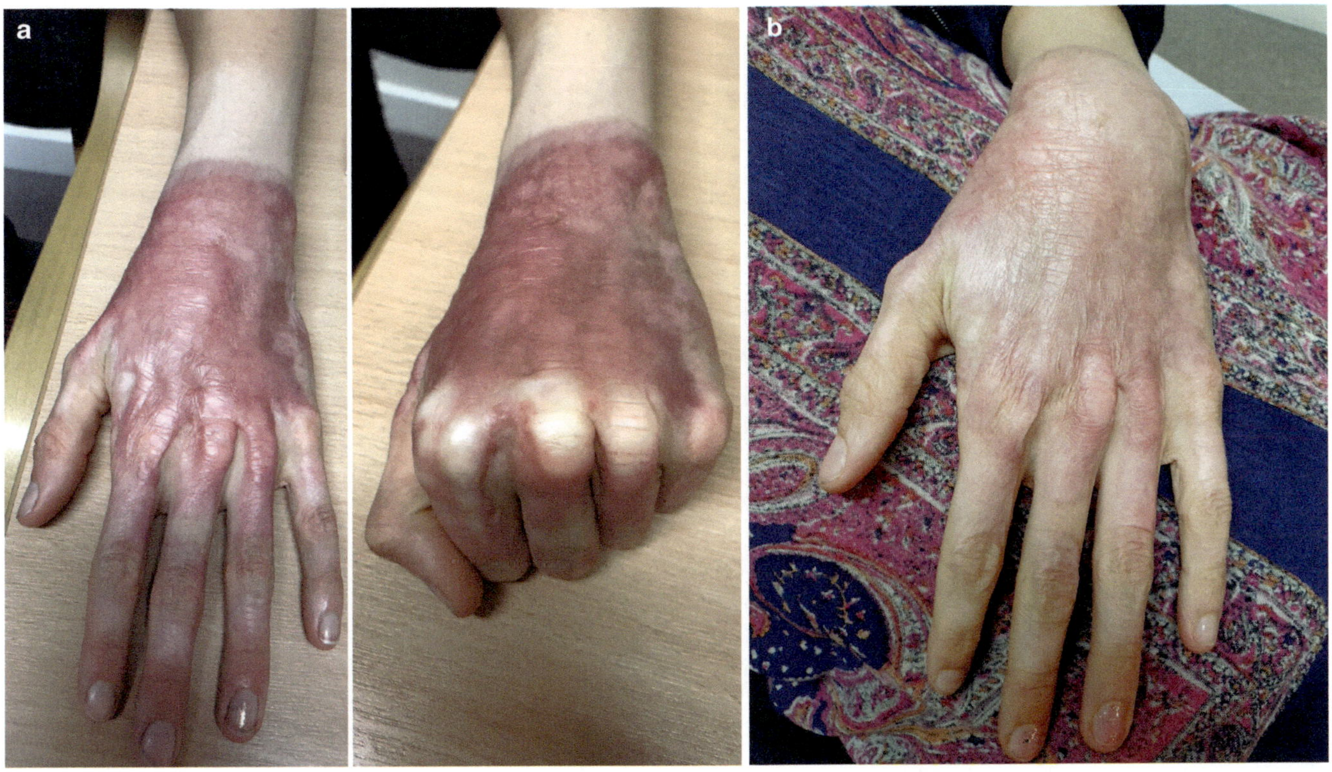

Fig. 9 (**a**) Extensive hypertrophic burn scars to the hands prior to four sessions of weekly Nd:YAG laser treatment. (**b**) Extensive hypertrophic burn scars to the hands after four sessions of weekly Nd:YAG laser treatment showing substantial reduction in erythema

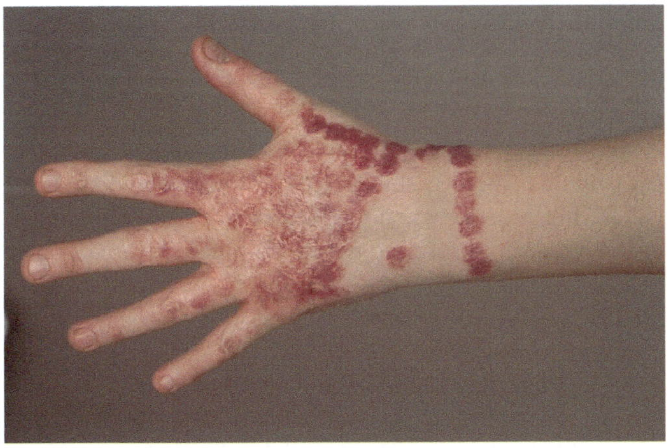

Fig. 10 Example of temporary pulsed dye laser purpuric skin changes which typically resolve after a few days. These can be expected with low pulse durations between 0.5 and 6 ms at modest to high energies

stay of treatment, often depending on availability. As a general rule, the Nd:YAG is preferred for visible vessels and the pulsed dye laser for generalised erythema but either laser is more than capable of dealing with this problem. Figure 11 demonstrates an example of severe burn scar erythema with extensive telangiectasia. Figure 12 demonstrates the long-pulsed Nd:YAG laser successfully treating an identified 'feeder' vessel.

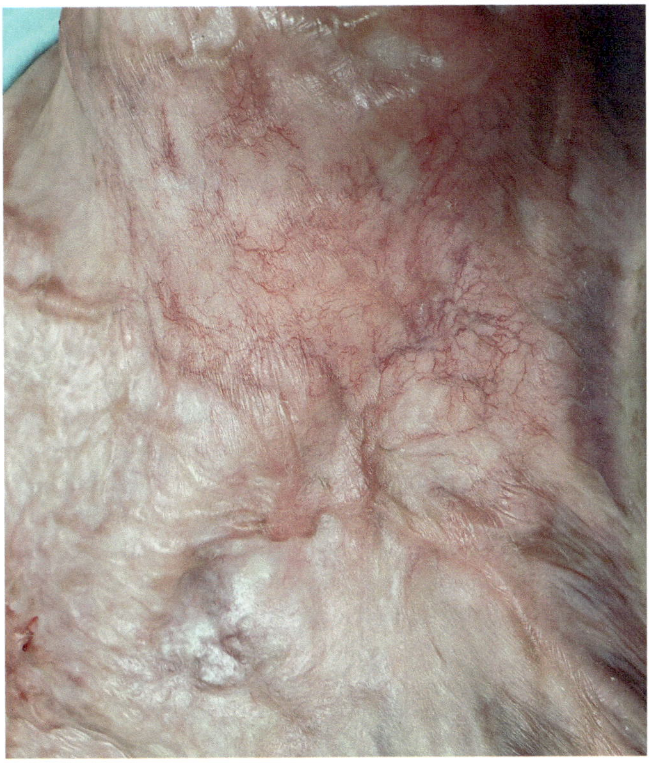

Fig. 11 Severe telangiectasia from burns scars affecting most of the body, in this case the neck and chest. Combined pulsed dye and Nd:YAG laser treatments are likely to afford most benefit

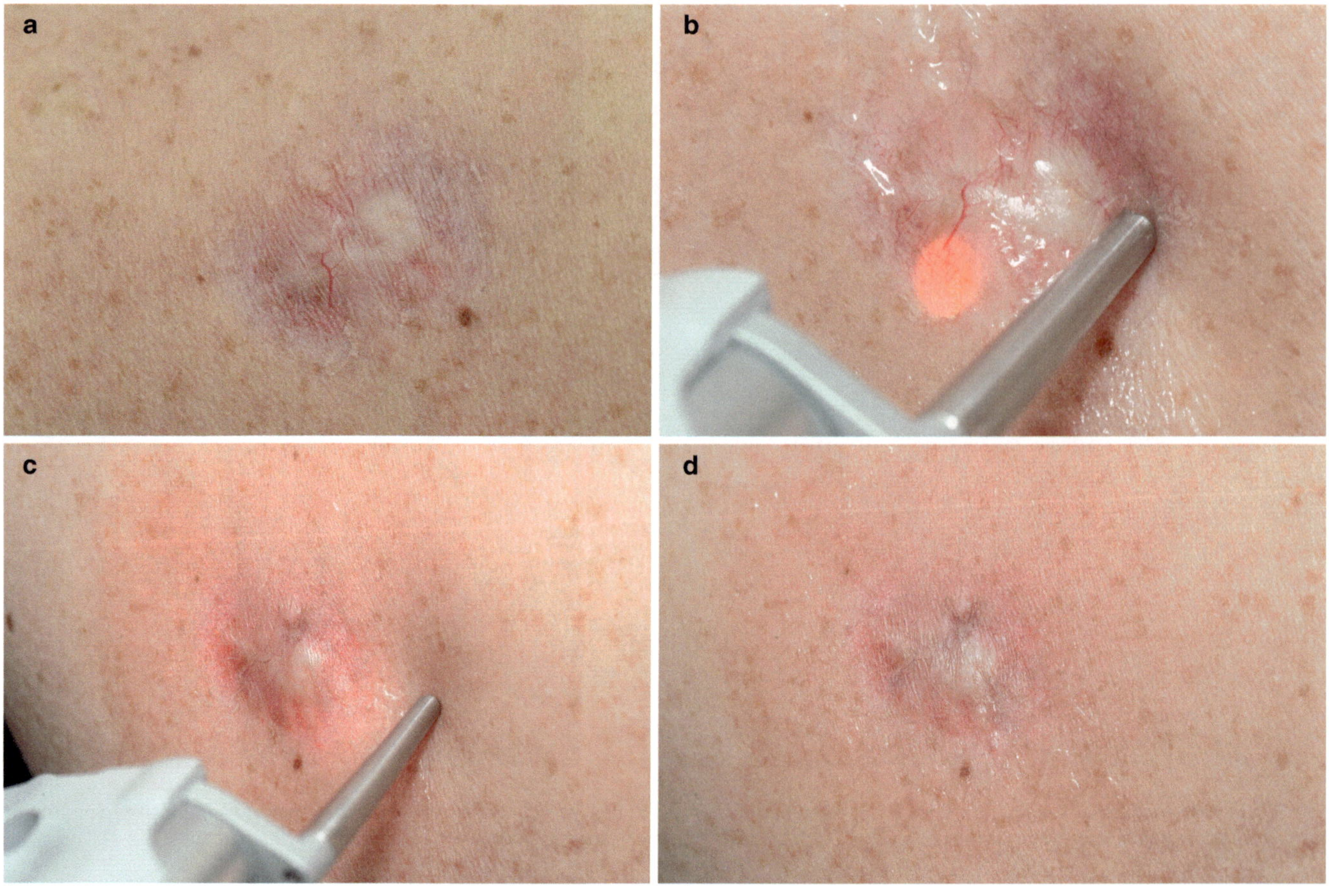

Fig. 12 (**a**) Telangiectasia in an area of previous keloid scarring after successful treatment with intralesional corticosteroid injections. (**b**) Nd:YAG laser with 5 mm spot size positioned with aiming beam over visible intradermal vessel with ultrasound gel and air cooling being administered. (**c**) Vessels visibly disappear during the course of the treatment. (**d**) Complete clearance of the telangiectasia by the end of the treatment lasting only a few seconds. Residual erythema associated with the treatment itself is to be expected

6.1 Summary (Vascular Laser Treatments for Scars)

The pulsed dye laser and Nd:YAG laser have a good track record in scar management, with the pulsed dye laser having the longest track record of any laser in scar management. Scar erythema, telangiectasia as especially amenable to treatment with these lasers. A course of treatment will typically be a minimum of six sessions but for large surface areas scars can be numerous treatments over the course of more than a year. Treatment intervals for small scars will typically be monthly, but for larger or more extensive scarring, very regular treatments will be required due to the numerous treatments required to cover wider larger areas if any tangible improvements are to be seen.

7 Keloid Scars

The first thing to bear in mind when considering treatment of any patient who has a keloid scar is this: 'what is the potential to cause scarring and hence keloid scarring with use of a laser on this patients' skin?' A lack of understanding of the underlying pathology and the incorrect or inappropriate use of lasers in keloid-forming patients can have severe negative consequences.

7.1 Vascular Lasers for Keloids

It is unlikely that vascular lasers by themselves can successfully treat keloid scars. Such lasers can be useful adjuncts to help with scar erythema and the consequences of multimodal treatment (such as resultant erythema and telangiectasia), which are commonly seen following intralesional injections or (for instance) radiotherapy (see Figs. 12 and 13).

Due to the nature of keloid scars, they are notoriously difficult to treat and have high rates of recurrence, and most patients referred for laser treatment will have had or be undertaking other treatment modalities concurrently. Some keloids are better treated by modalities other than laser (Fig. 14).

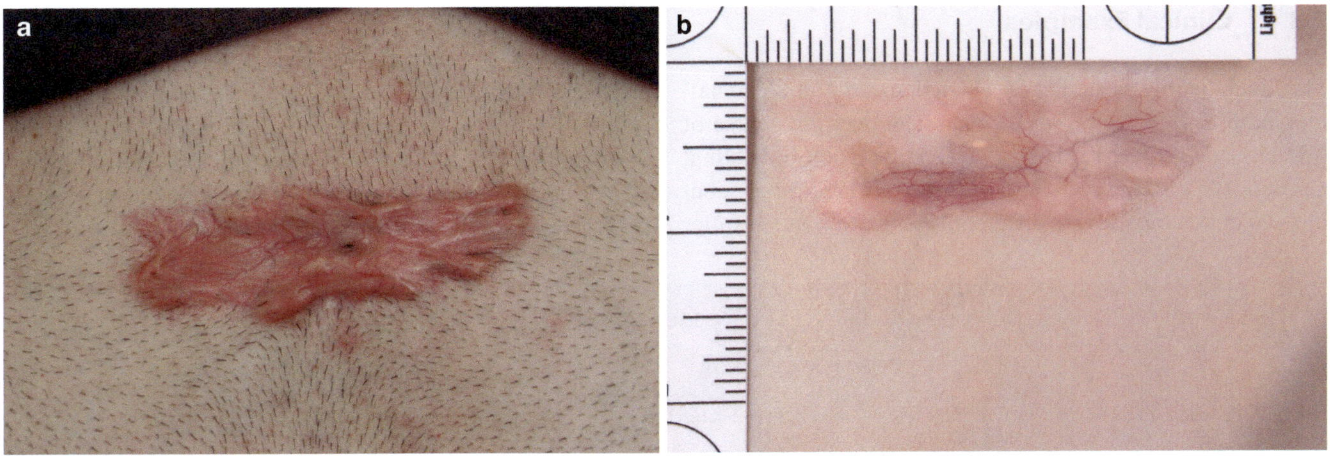

Fig. 13 (**a**) A classic chest keloid scar that has been partially responsive to intralesional steroid injections and for which vascular laser treatment can offer improvements in relation to telangiectasia, erythema, and pruritis. Folliculitis can be a cause or perpetuating factor for these lesions, and depilation is an under-utilised modality for these patients. (**b**) Another example of classical post-steroid-injection keloid scar changes susceptible to vascular laser treatment

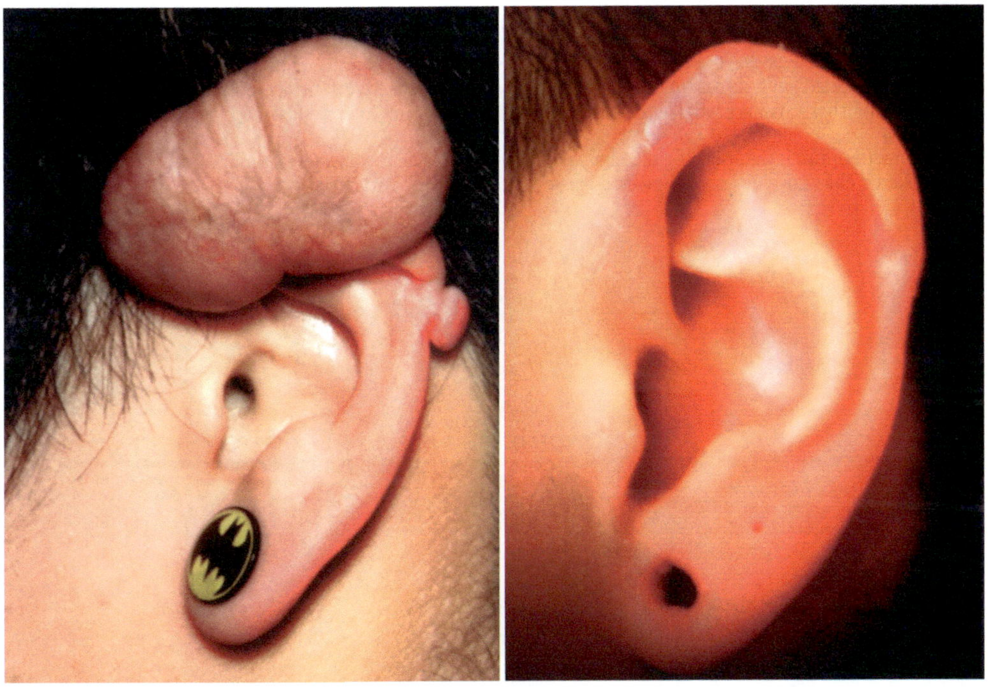

Fig. 14 This patient of the senior author had surgical excision and reconstruction of the ear and a single postoperative intralesional steroid injection without recurrence for a number of years prior to discharge from surveillance. Lasers are not a panacea

7.2 Ablative Lasers for Keloids

Keloid scars must therefore be considered a chronic disease, and more importantly any treatment given must not be considered in isolation, but as part of a tailored treatment plan—which by default must include intralesional treatments if success is to be achieved.

Early, regular and aggressive treatment of keloid scars with intralesional corticosteroid treatment is one of the simplest and best chances of improvement and resolution of these scars. Similarly, most modalities that are more invasive will often rely on adjunctive use of corticosteroids to limit the potential for recurrence.

One of the most significant ways that laser treatment can help with keloid scars is to make recalcitrant scars more amenable to conventional and ancillary treatment. Hence a significant portion of keloid scars referred for laser are referred as those ‘unresponsive to intralesional corticosteroids’. This may well be the case, but more often than not, the amount and dose of steroid used, frequency of delivery, and tolerance of the patient to painful injections are actually the limiting factors. Furthermore, there is a distinct category of keloid scars that are more recalcitrant to treatment, and these are very stiff and hard keloids into which it is very difficult to administer steroid injections. It is with this type of scar that there is perhaps the greatest mileage with ablative carbon dioxide laser treatment:

7.3 Clinical Examples

The thick keloid scar that is ablated in an 'intralesional' manner using the CO_2 laser tends to heal over the course of 3 weeks or so (Figs. 15, 16, and 17). At the point of healing, a proportion of these scars will show signs of recurrence, but the scar characteristics are different, and they are much softer and amenable to/responsive to intralesional treatment. Hence, the CO_2 laser presents the opportunity to achieve a number of positive outcomes for patients with keloid scars as follows:

1. Immediacy of result. Patients can often be tearful as they see an immediate improvement and a flat scar, possibly for the first time in many years.

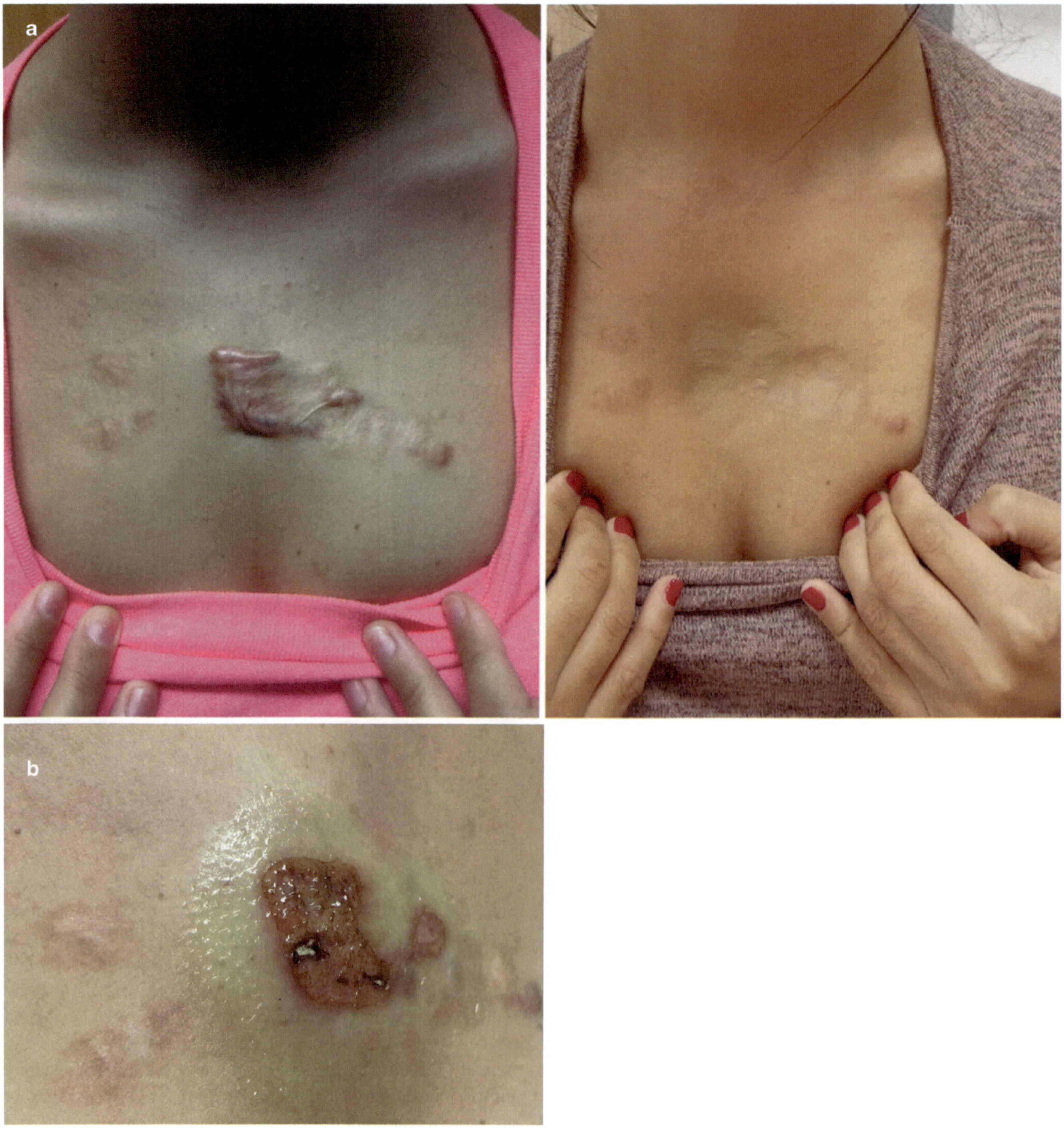

Fig. 15 (**a**) Keloid scar before and after carbon dioxide laser ablation resulting in a scar that can for the first time be covered with cosmetic camouflage. Small areas of recurrence can easily be maintained with further corticosteroid injections. In this case, only one small area of the scar requires occasional regular maintenance injections 3 years after ablative laser treatment. The scar was prominent and generally unresponsive to any treatment for the preceding 4 years before laser treatment. (**b**) Chest keloid immediately after ablation with carbon dioxide laser

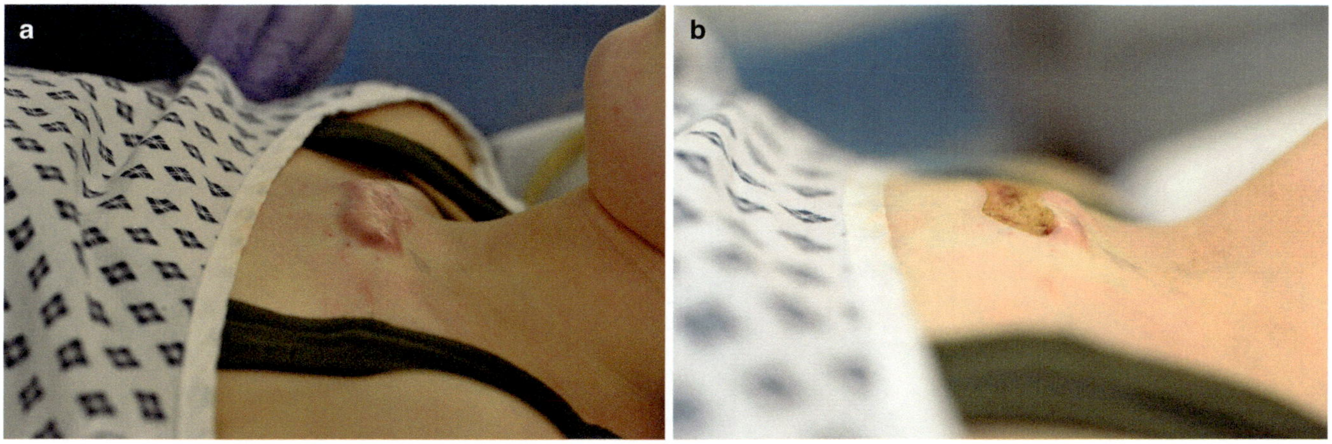

Fig. 16 (**a**) Chest keloid scar immediately prior to ablative CO_2 laser. (**b**) Chest keloid midway through ablative CO_2 laser treatment

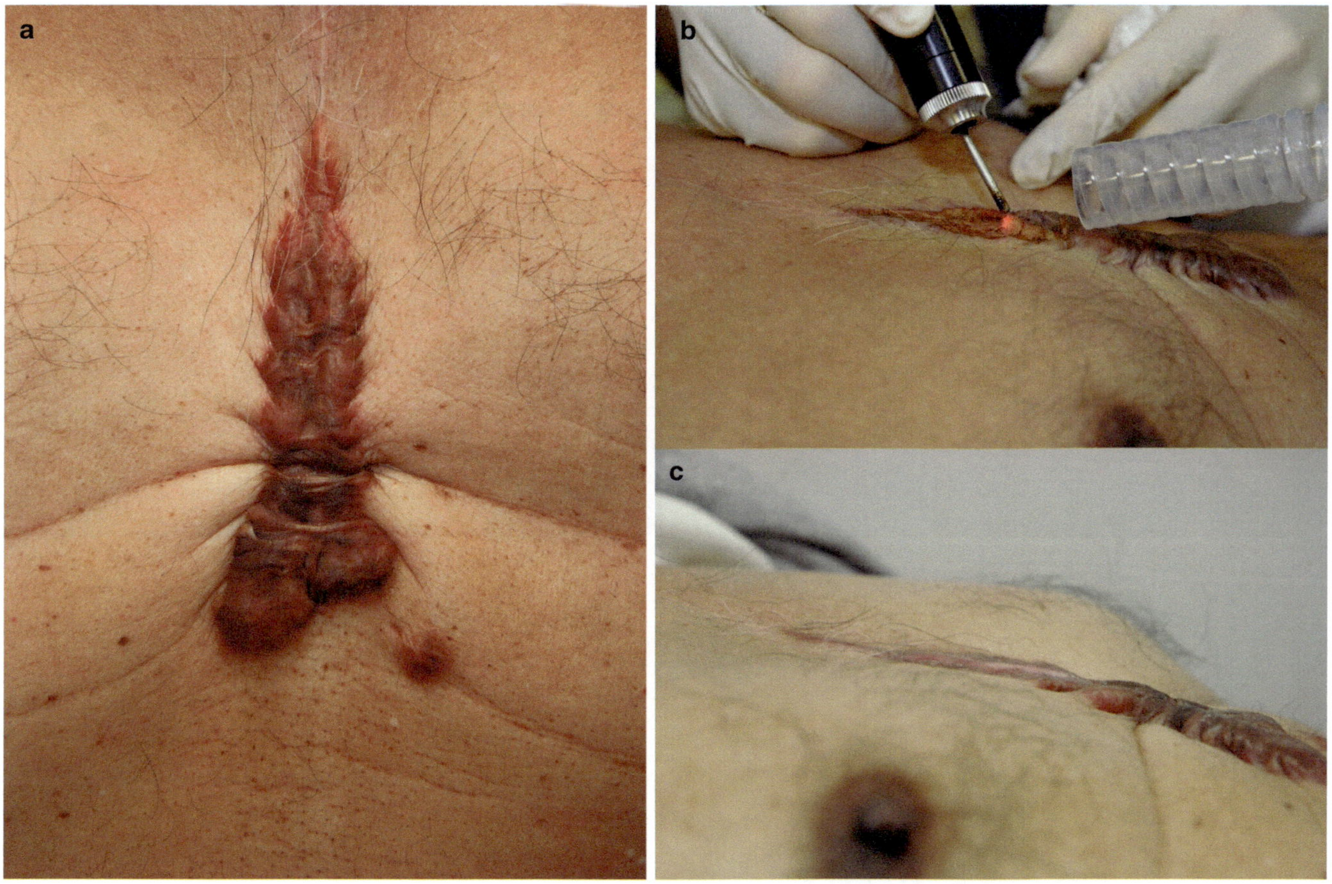

Fig. 17 (**a**) Extremely stiff and recalcitrant keloid scar present for greater than 7 years in a patient with skin type/ethnicity 4. Cicatrisation is causing deep skin rhytids. The scar is so stiff that it is difficult to penetrate with a needle and to turgid to infiltrate sufficient quantities of therapeutic intralesional corticosteroid. (**b**) Carbon dioxide laser intralesional ablation of the upper half of the scar under local anaesthesia. (**c**) Healed area of scar remains flat some months after treatment and has not recurred. Carbon dioxide laser intralesional ablation of 50% of scar under local anaesthesia. (**d**) Completion of ablative laser treatment at 5 weeks and at 6 months after treatment showing a flat scar for the first time in very many years. (**e**) Final result. A small area of recurrence in the central portion only has required repeat steroid injections. It is unknown what makes some areas and not others prone to recurrence. These recurrent areas are soft and amenable to corticosteroid maintenance treatment, whereas the size and stiffness of the pretreatment scar was not amenable to treatment

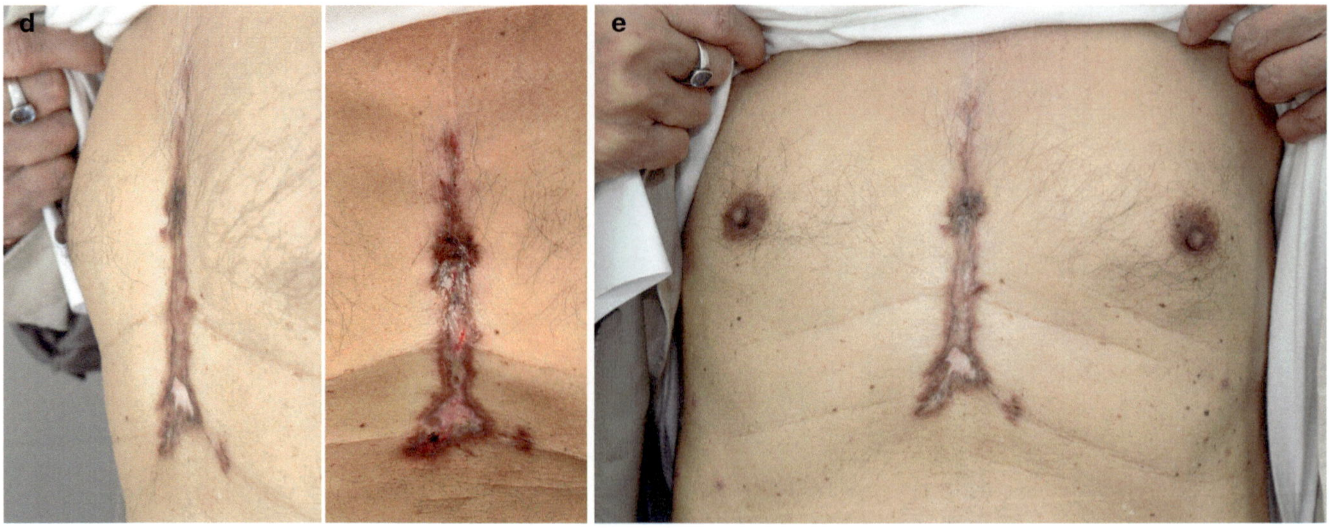

Fig.17 contiuned

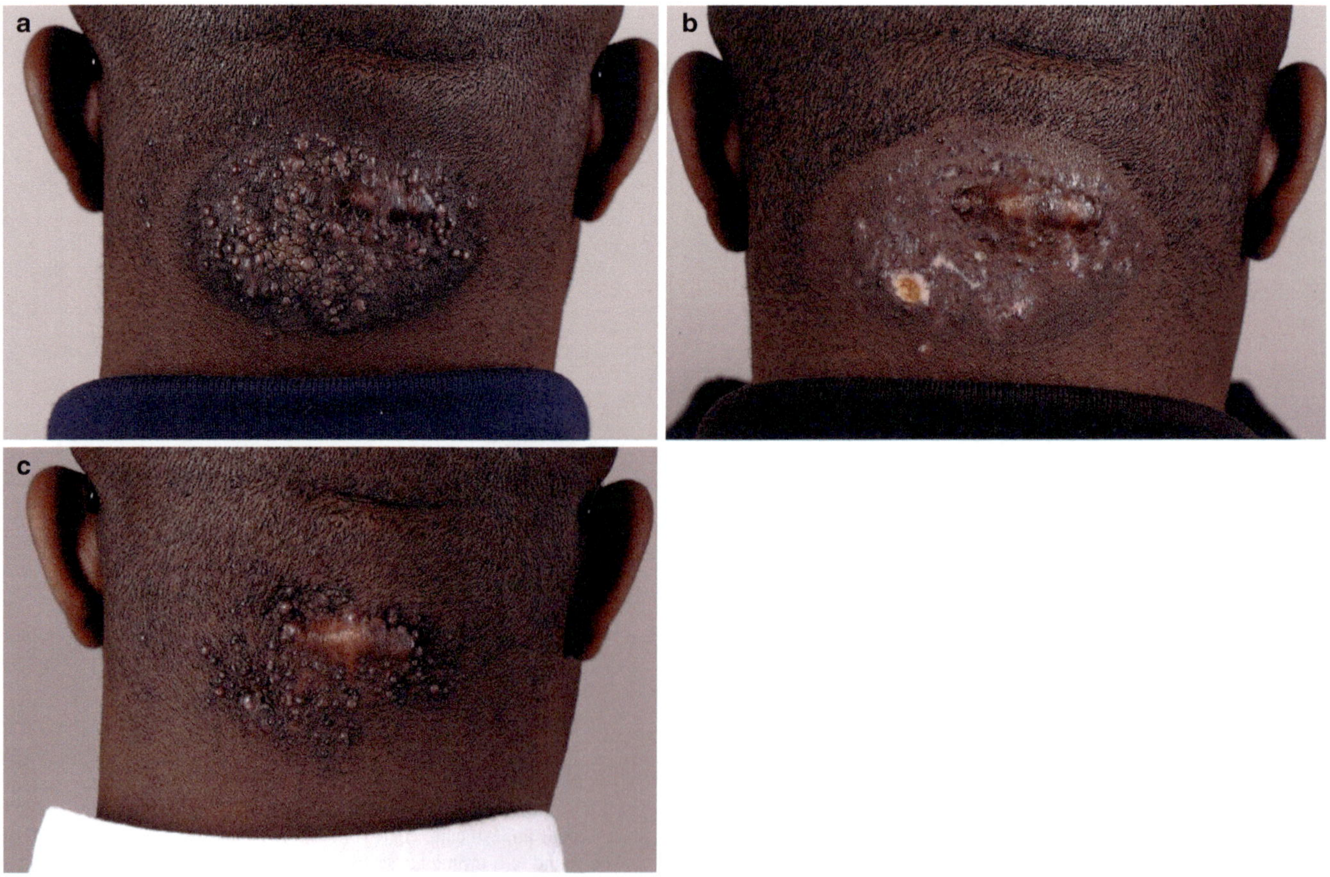

Fig. 18 (**a**) Complex keloid folliculitis is caused by/perpetuated by hair and is very difficult to treat. It is common in face, neck, and beard areas. (**b**) A single session of carbon dioxide laser ablation has cleared a substantial proportion of the keloid scars and had a significant positive impact on the folliculitis and underlying hair follicles. A substantial reduction in the bulk of any keloid assists any and all ancillary measures in the ability to control the keloid scarring and in particular its gradual progression. (**c**) Some months later, there are some areas of recurrence, but the overall burden of keloid is much less, and the keloids that exist are more susceptible and responsive to intra-lesion treatments, which are also more feasible and better tolerated. Patients are far happier about their condition as they can see, often for the first time, tangible improvements

2. A scar that heals flat and can be covered with cosmetic camouflage, often for the first time.
3. A scar that, even if recurrent, is thereafter manageable with maintenance intralesional steroid injections—where previously this was not achievable.

Keloid scars are commonly a consequence of, or perpetuated by, folliculitis. Keloid scar folliculitis is a condition that has not been described in detail as a clinical entity. The underlying causative or perpetuating factor is hair, and treatment of the hair is essential if success is to be achieved with the keloid scarring.

Figure 18 demonstrates a case of complex keloid scar folliculitis successfully treated with CO_2 laser in a manner whereby the keloids and individual hair follicles are ablated as far as is feasible. Laser depilation is especially difficult along conventional lines in patients with skin type 5 or 6 with scar folliculitis/keloids, and the ability of conventional non-ablative lasers to successfully treat the hair follicles is limited.

The role of fractional laser in the treatment of keloids is uncertain.

Not all keloid scars are suitable for laser treatment (Fig. 19), and there is sometimes a role for surgery as in this example.

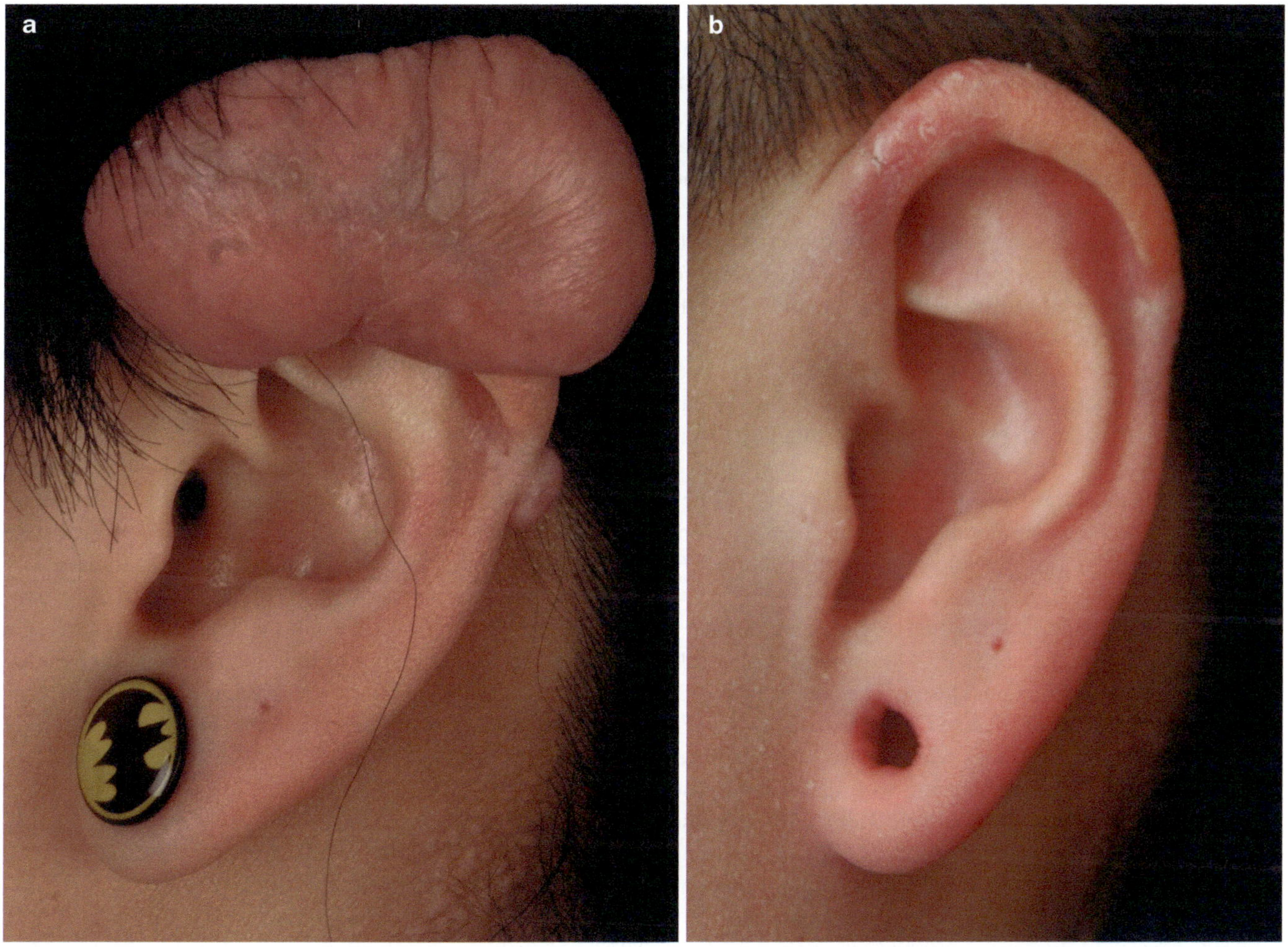

Fig. 19 (**a**) One large (superior) and one small (lateral) areas of keloid scarring of the ear. Surgery is often the method that provides the most immediate and impactful results in the context of a holistic management regime that includes pressure clips and intralesional steroids to limit recurrence potential which is up to 50%. Due to the immediacy and quality of the result and the rapid healing time, surgery of this nature is preferred to other treatments such as laser, intralesional cryotherapy, and other modalities in this anatomical location. (**b**) Patient 6 weeks after a single surgical excision of keloid scars from the ear. Surprisingly, only a single intraoperative steroid injection was required and the patient has now been recurrence-free for over 5 years

8 Hypertrophic Scars and Contour

Many scars present contour irregularities which can be amenable to laser treatment. The contouring of scars has traditionally remained in the domain of ablative lasers in either fractionated or ablative modes.

The carbon dioxide laser remains the most versatile and powerful laser modality to allow for the greatest impact on scar contours and work best in scars that are mature. Patients describe benefits from more supple scars, improved appearances and in our experience a tangible change in their ability to cover their scars with make-up or camouflage.

8.1 Ablative CO_2 Laser

Figure 20 demonstrates a recalcitrant hypertrophic facial burn scar that has been treated (a–d, right cheek) with a combination of carbon dioxide laser and intralesional steroid injection and which for the first time has resulted in a flattened scar which can be concealed with make-up. The immediacy of such treatments, often after a single treatment, in patients with long-standing scars is very powerful in the positive psychological impact that can be achieved for patients. Contouring of skin grafts is also possible with the ablative laser at modest depth (Fig. 20e, f).

A common problem after meshed skin grafts have been used for reconstruction, typically after burns, is the residual mesh pattern. These mesh patterns are very difficult to treat, and deep/ingrained mesh patterns are only amenable to minor improvements at best. The best opportunity to help mesh patterns that are considerably raised and constitute epidermal and partial dermal thickness is with the ablative CO_2 laser as illustrated in Fig. 20.

For thickened mature scars that would benefit from a reduction in profile, the ablative CO_2 laser still has a role, despite the advent of fractional lasers. The patient in Fig. 21 received three sessions of ablative CO_2 laser to the prominent scarring of the nasolabial areas which subsequently allowed her to conceal much of her scarring with make-up—something she could not previously achieve. Her smile has subsequently been far less impacted by abnormal contour of her nasolabial folds and she has been delighted with the outcome (Fig. 22).

8.2 Laser Resurfacing

Fractional carbon dioxide laser resurfacing has encountered a number of iterations since its initial entry to the market. Conventionally, fractional resurfacing acted at the epidermal and superficial dermal level removing precisely islands of skin whilst preserving others in a distribution and pattern set by the practitioner via a computer pattern generator (CPG). More modern versions of these lasers now (often in concert) allow for deeply penetrating laser energy delivery into the deeper dermis, typically with much narrower beams, and the evidence is that this promotes collagen remodelling at a physiological level at this depth, and with a more enduring impact.

Whilst it is important not to overstate the impact that laser resurfacing can make, either cosmetically or for scar management, it remains one of the most useful modalities for a range of scar problems including:

- Scar contour (and hence camouflagability of scars).
- Tension in scars and mild scar contracture.
- General skin condition.
- Pigmentation.

It is always recommended to undertake test patching to ascertain the most appropriate laser settings (for safety but also efficacy) and, if possible, to achieve a combination of superficial resurfacing and more deeply penetrating laser treatment.

Figures 23 and 24 demonstrate the significant impact of general skin condition and camouflagability of facial burn scars after sessions of deep CO_2 laser resurfacing at high density using medium energies.

8.3 Summary: Ablative and Fractional Laser for Scars

Of the main ablative lasers (erbium:YAG and carbon dioxide laser), the CO_2 laser is more versatile and effective in general terms. Ablative lasers can improve scar contour, deal with complex problems including keloids, and help to generally improve the smoothness of the skin. Patients invariably comment about the improvements in the smoothness of the skin and their increased ability to hide their scars with make-up after treatment. There is as yet no 'camouflagability' outcome measure after scar interventions, but it is an important outcome for most patients.

9 Laser Depilation for Scar Folliculitis and Heterotopic Hair Growth

The use of lasers for depilation is well recognised and has spawned a huge industry in the aesthetic sector. So long as hairs still have their colour, i.e. are yet to turn grey, an effective reduction can be achieved using laser treatment (multiple sessions are required). The alexandrite 755 nm and diode lasers have demonstrated excellent outcomes in hair removal due to its longer wavelength allowing deeper penetration into the skin, therefore destroying the hair follicles at their root.

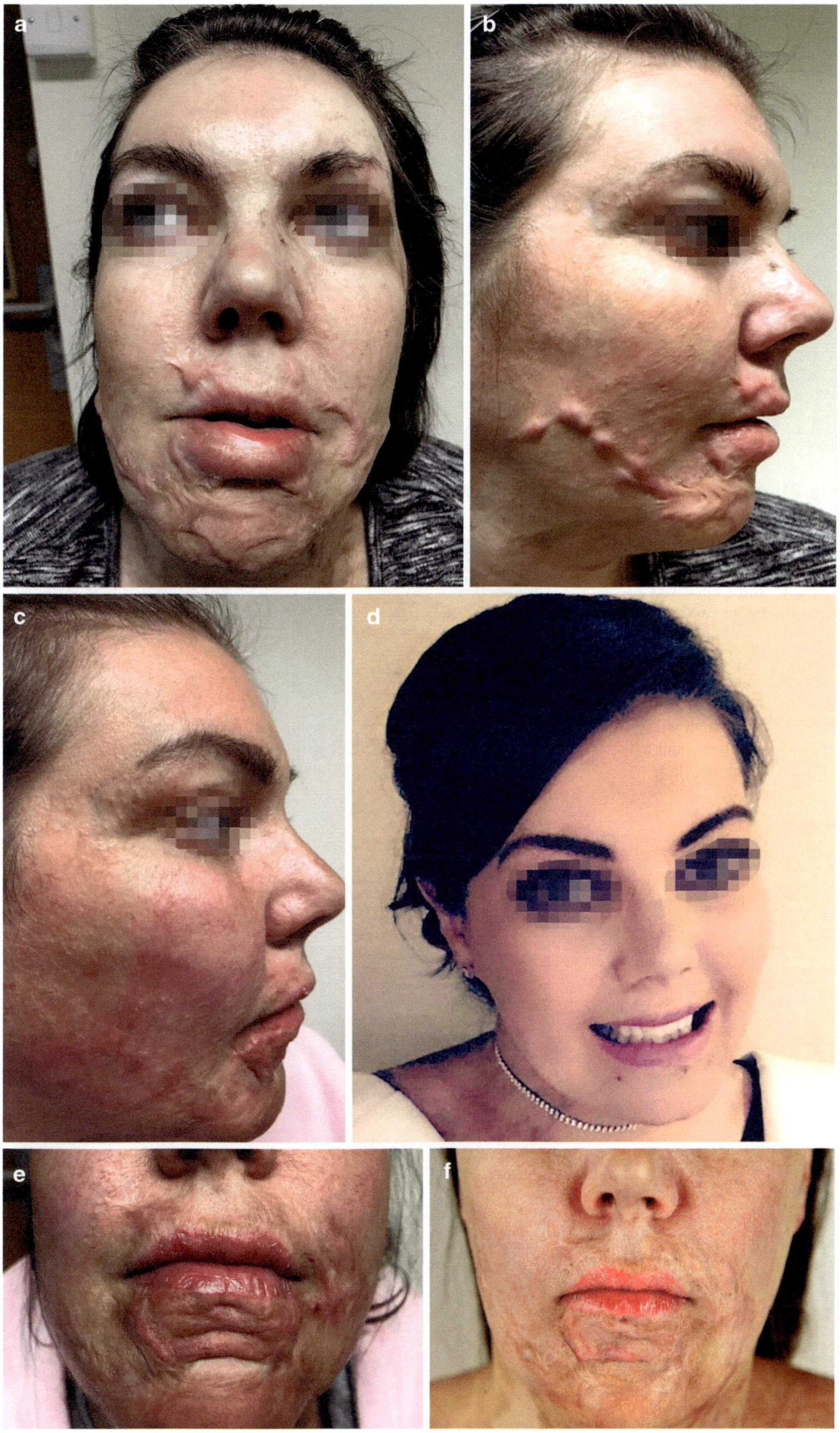

Fig. 20 (**a**) Extensive facial hypertrophic burn scars. (**b**) Hypertrophic burn scars on the right side of the cheek prior to treatment. (**c**) Hypertrophic burn scars on the right side of the cheek after ablative carbon dioxide laser and a single intralesional corticosteroid injection. (**d**) One of the most impactful outcomes from laser treatment along with ancillary modalities is the ability to conceal more of the scarring with cosmetic camouflage or lighter make-up. Any and all scar treatments must be in the context of ancillary measures and personal/lifestyle factors. (**e**) A full-thickness skin graft of the lower lip by the treating surgeon in the burns unit has very successfully treated the lower lip eversion. However, the patient complained of bulkiness of the graft. (**f**) A bulky full-thickness skin graft has become less bulky after a session of CO_2 laser ablation. The laser allows for very fine contouring in a bloodless field in a tissue-sparing manner

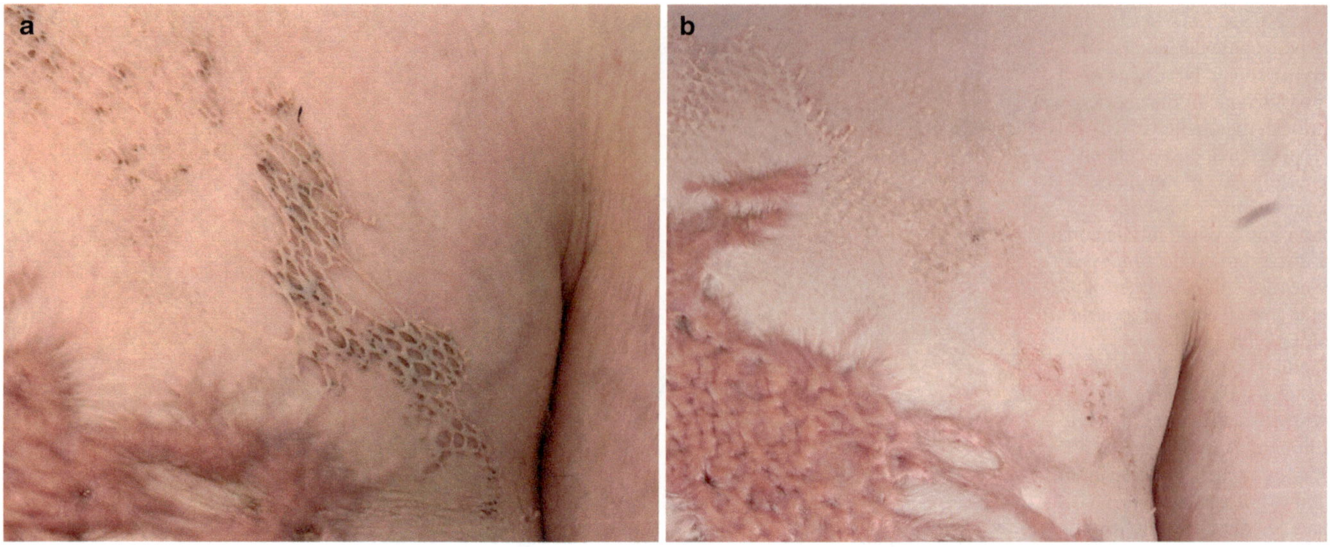

Fig. 21 (**a**) Mesh pattern of skin graft prior to ablative CO_2 laser treatment. (**b**) Mesh pattern of skin graft after ablative CO_2 laser treatment

Fig. 22 (**a**) Patient with extensive burn scars before and after three ablative CO_2 laser treatment sessions to the nasolabial and nasojugal folds. (**b**) A close up of the areas of thickened but mature scarring that can be successfully treated with ablative laser treatment to allow better camouflage

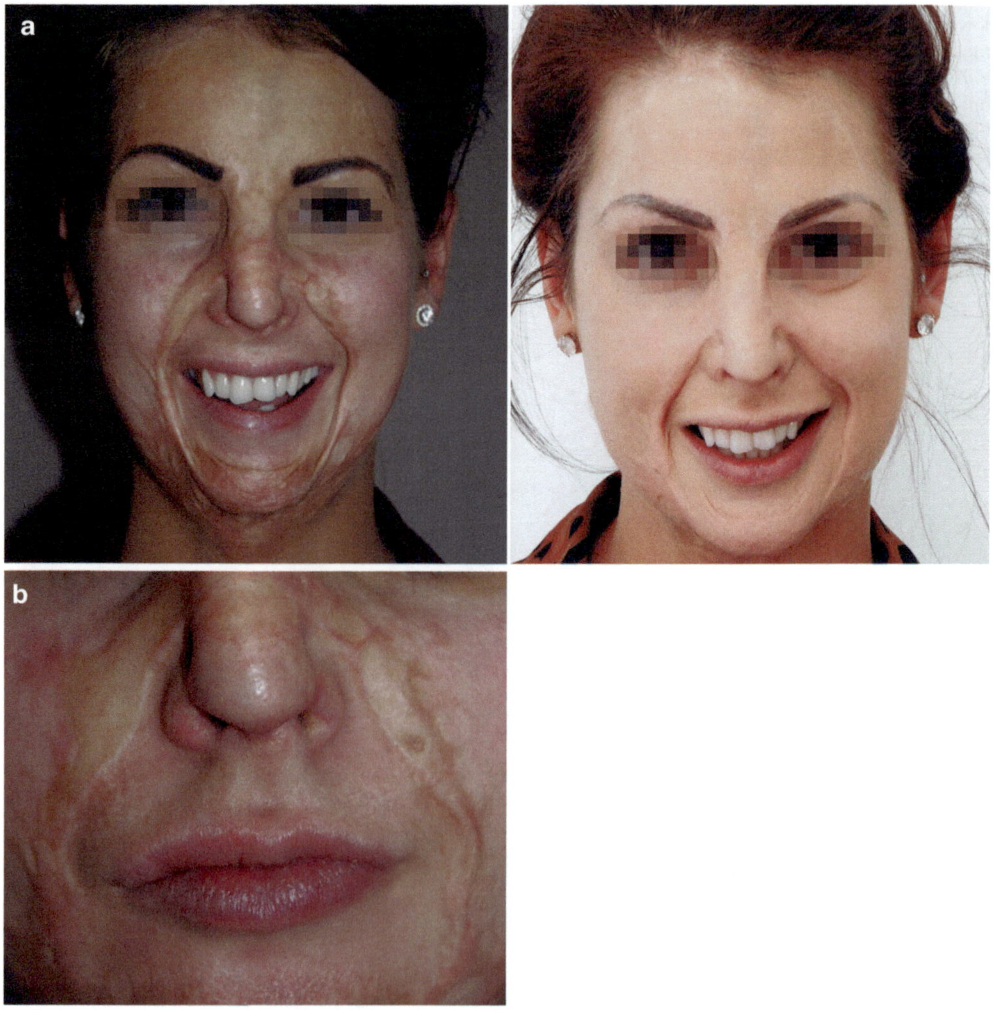

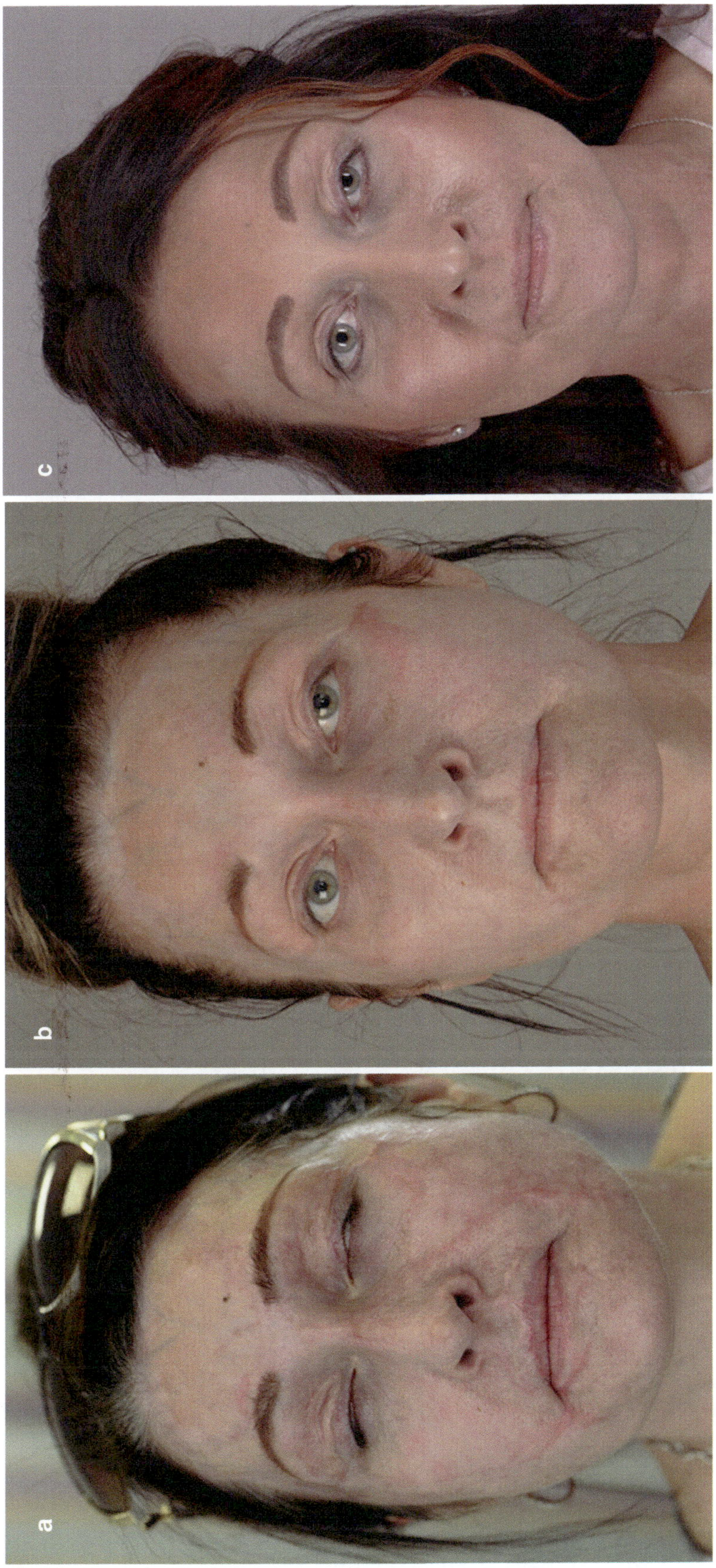

Fig. 23 (**a**) Facial burn scars after an assault prior to treatment. (**b**) Facial burn scars after two sessions of fractional CO_2 laser deep resurfacing using Lumenis UltraPulse laser (without make-up). (**c**) Facial burn scars after two sessions of fractional CO_2 laser deep resurfacing using Lumenis UltraPulse laser (with make-up)

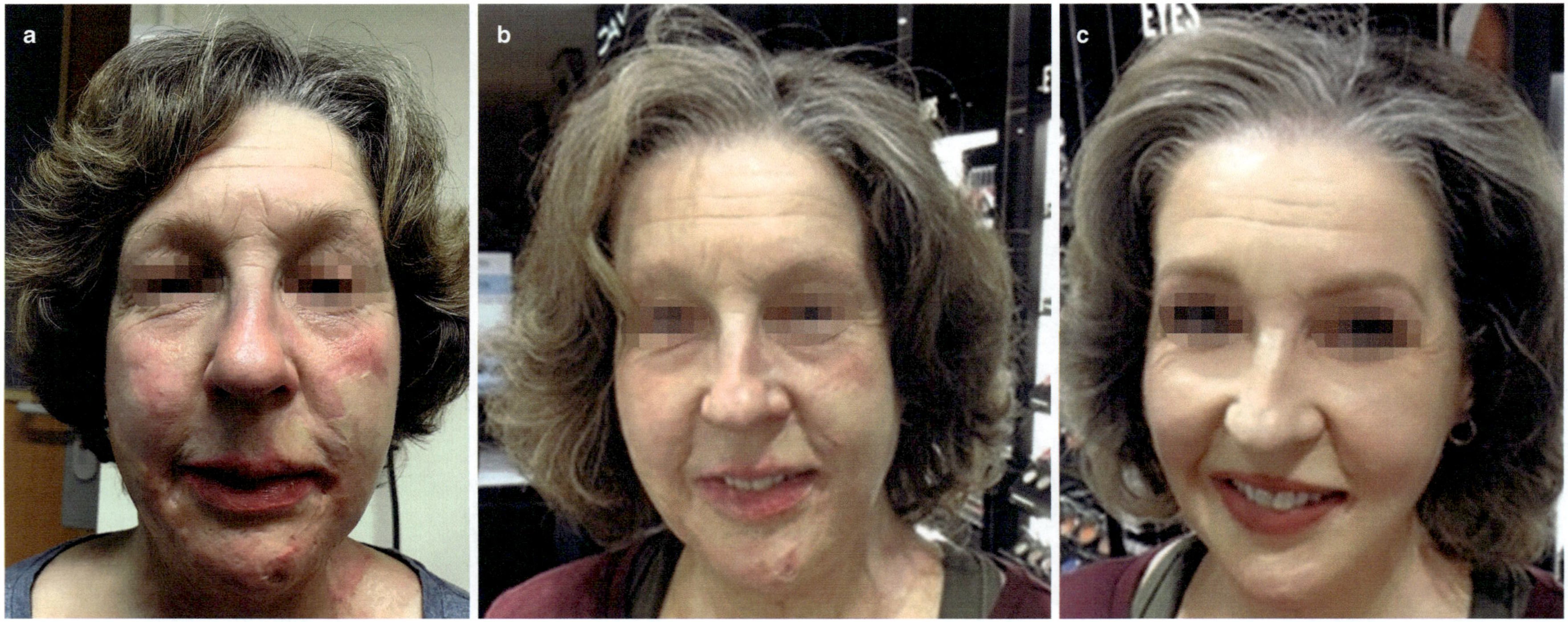

Fig. 24 (**a**) Facial burn scars before one session of fractional CO_2 laser deep resurfacing using Lumenis AcuPulse laser. (**b**) Facial burn scars after one session of fractional CO_2 laser deep resurfacing using Lumenis AcuPulse laser. (**c**) Facial burn scars after one session of fractional CO_2 laser deep resurfacing using Lumenis AcuPulse laser (after a makeover with high-street cosmetics)

We have used the alexandrite laser with air cooling as well as the diode laser with contact cooling with equal success for depilation in scar tissue.

Hair is most effectively treated with laser when the skin type is pale (Fitzpatrick types 1–2) whilst the hair is dark. The darker the skin or the lighter the hair, the less effective or more challenging the treatment.

Scar folliculitis is, surprisingly, not a widely recognised problem, despite it being one of the most frequently encountered problems for patients with scars. Folliculitis itself can also be the primary underlying pathology that causes and perpetuates keloid scarring, especially in patients with Fitzpatrick skin types 5 and 6 (Fig. 18). Hence, laser depilation plays an important role in the management of patients with scars.

The most severe types of scar folliculitis occur in skin types V–VI, and laser depilation is not typically useful in these severe cases, and new approaches and interventions are required (Figs. 25, 26, and 27).

Complex keloid scar folliculitis in type 5–6 skin is a complex and difficult problem to treat. However, it can be successfully addressed with the help of laser treatment that can ablate the nodules of keloid scar including the hair follicles as demonstrated in Fig. 18. Radiotherapy may also play an important role in the management of this condition.

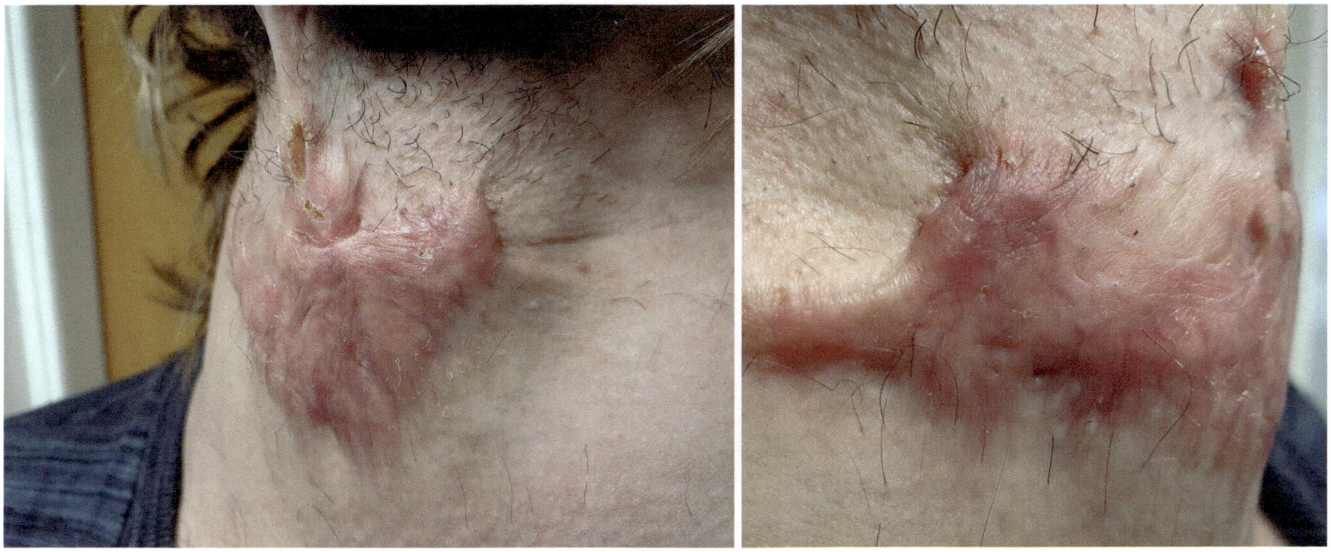

Fig. 25 Scar folliculitis of the pre-tracheal area of the neck with close up

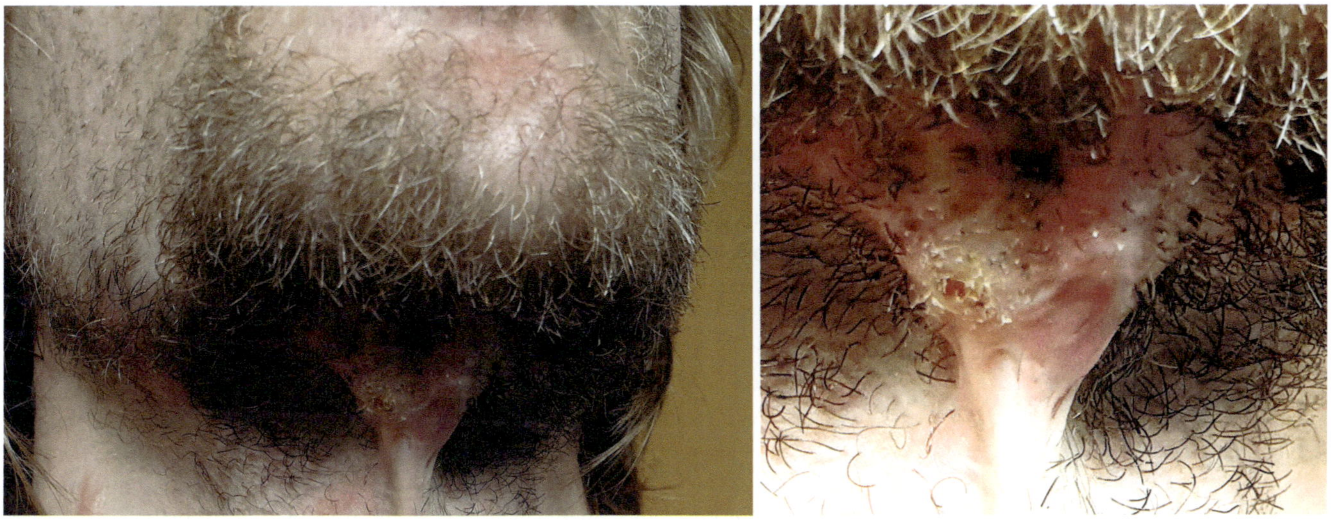

Fig. 26 Scar folliculitis in the area between the chin and neck. Regular depilation will lead to considerable symptomatic improvements

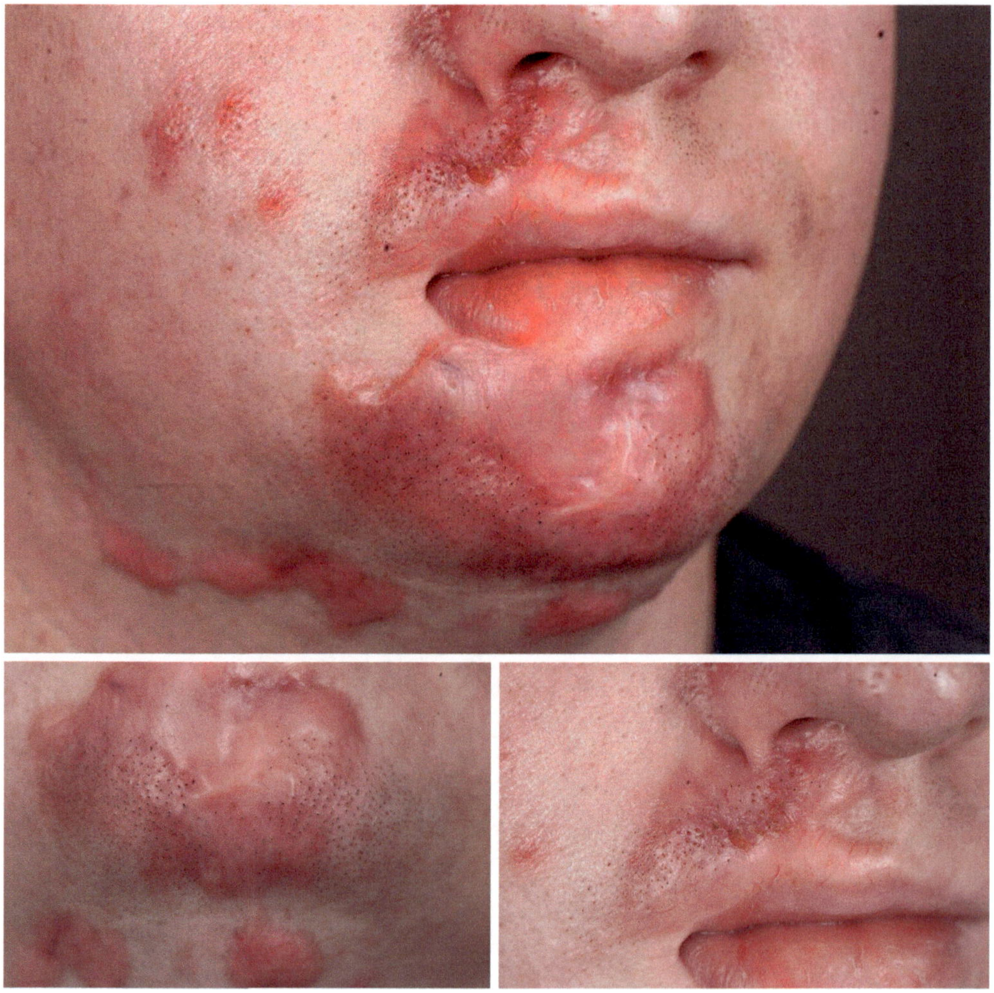

Fig. 27 Classical hypertrophic scar folliculitis. Tends to respond well to conventional laser depilation, with increased success with more frequent treatment (such as weekly). Furthermore, if vascular lasers are being used for hypertrophic scarring and erythema, Nd:YAG laser can have a combined effect to treat both vascularity and an additional (secondary) depilatory effect

10 Acne Scarring

Cosmetic camouflage remains the mainstay of treatment for acne scarring. This is less acceptable to men compared with women, and the sexes (in general terms) have different perspectives on what is a successful outcome from treatment because for most women if the scars can be covered with make-up then this is a success, but for most men an outcome in the absence of any camouflage is the expectation. Fractional laser treatment offers one of most effective treatments to treat atrophic acne scars, but it is important not to inappropriately raise the expectation of patients. Figure 28 provides an example of what can be achieved, and readers are referred to the separate chapter in this book on acne scarring.

11 Summary

The choice of laser as well as laser parameters is crucial in order to provide the best patient outcomes. Due to increased public awareness, patients actively seek out laser treatments and will travel far; however, this can create logistical challenges for treatments that require test patching and multiple sessions and has significant cost implications. Through an increase in referrals, we have found ourselves acting as a quaternary referral centre spanning a substantial part of the UK. There is increasing evidence that a variety of scars can be improved with a range of laser treatments, but the field continues to develop. Laser management of burns scars is highly specialised. A great deal of work is needed in relation to objective outcome measures in this area. Even within a supra-regional service, patient numbers, outcomes, multiple variables, and simultaneous combination treatments make objective evaluation and research very challenging—mirroring many other areas of scar and burns practice. This is compounded further by the variability of lasers and brands which are all different according to manufacturer, and features upon which brands are keen to promote variance for both clinical and marketing purposes. Well-selected and compliant patients with burns and complex scars may benefit from a range of interventions using lasers. The clinical and research challenges

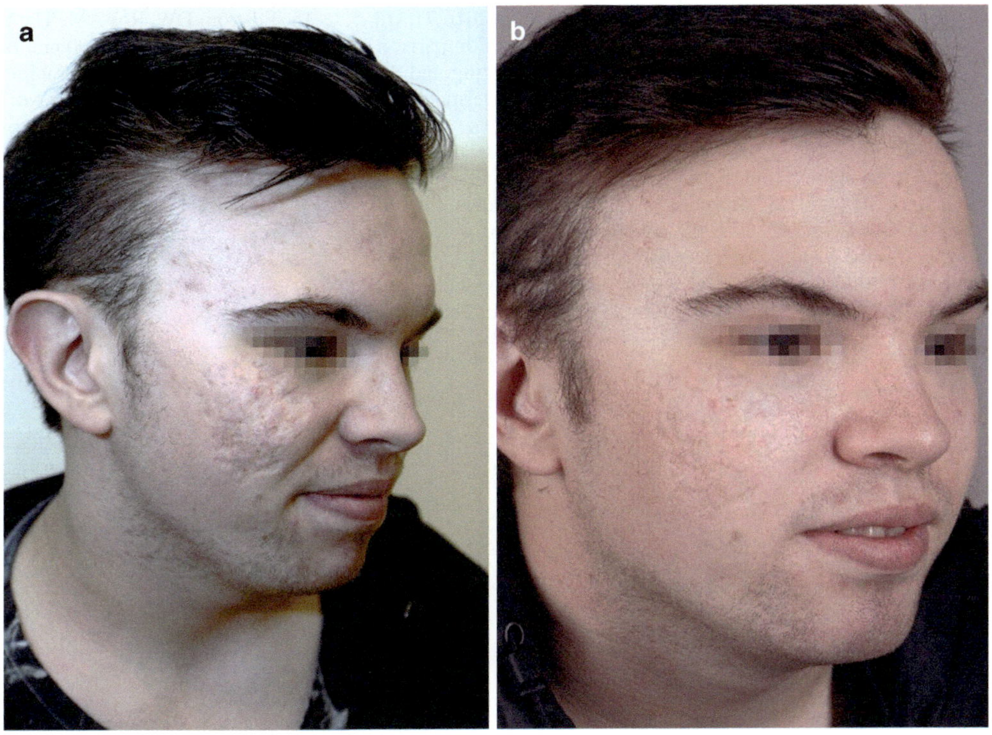

Fig. 28 (**a**) Patient with a combination of acne scarring and previous vascular malformation of the right cheek prior to treatment with three sessions of fractional laser resurfacing. (**b**) Patient with a combination of acne scarring and previous vascular malformation of the right cheek after three sessions of fractional laser resurfacing

of this work are enormous and at present we have to rely mostly on clinical subjective evaluation and most importantly on direct patient feedback. Elsewhere in this text are voluminous appraisals of the evidence base for laser scar practice.

All scars and patients are unique. A comprehensive laser service for managing scars relies on the availability of a wide range of laser modalities, the capital investment for which is large. The expense of lasers and their upkeep, and limited numbers of experienced practitioners due to relatively low numbers of a wide range of complex (especially burns) scars naturally lends itself to large laser centres with larger patient catchment areas. Whilst this has a potential negative effect on treatment accessibility for patients, this provides a platform for research and development, audit and much-needed work on outcome measures as well as focussing treatments in areas where there is sufficient expertise and multidisciplinary teams. The incorporation of laser treatment availability for patients in the 2018 UK National Burn Care Standards acknowledged for the first time the importance of this modality in scar management in the UK [5].

Acknowledgement A number of patients treated had their initial burn care in other hospitals around the country, not at the burn/laser centre of the senior author. Their excellent treatment prior to the commencement of laser treatment is acknowledged and applauded.

Note: All patients featured in this chapter underwent laser treatment or surgery under the care of Professor Shokrollahi and consent provided in writing for publication.

References

1. Gauglitz GG, Korting HC, Pavicic T, Ruzicka T, Jeschke MG. Hypertrophic scarring and keloids: pathomechanisms and current and emerging treatment strategies. Mol Med. 2011;17:113–25.
2. McGoldrick RB, Theodorakopoulou E, Azzopardi EA, Murison M. Lasers and ancillary treatments for scar management part 2: keloid, hypertrophic, pigmented and acne scars. Scars Burn Heal. 2017;3:2059513116689805. https://doi.org/10.1177/2059513116689805.
3. McGoldrick RB, Sawyer A, Davis CR, Theodorakopoulou E, Murison M. Lasers and ancillary treatments for scar management: personal experience over two decades and contextual review of the literature. Part I: burn scars. Scars Burn Heal. 2016;2:2059513116642090. https://doi.org/10.1177/2059513116642090.
4. Shokrollahi K, Linday KJ. Laser management of scars (Ch44). In: Whitaker, Shokrollahi, Dickson, editors. Oxford handbook of burns. Oxford: Oxford University Press; 2019.
5. British Burns Association Professional standards 2018 for adult and paediatric burn care. https://www.britishburnassociation.org/wpcontent/uploads/2018/11/BCSO-2018-FINAL-v28.pdf.
6. Haina D, Landthaler M, Braun-Falco O, Waidelich W. Comparison of the maximum coagulation depth in human skin for different types of medical lasers. Lasers Surg Med. 1987;7(4):355–62. https://doi.org/10.1002/lsm.1900070411.
7. Shokrollahi K, Raymond E, Murison MSC. Lasers: principles and surgical applications. J Surg. 2004;2:28–34. https://doi.org/10.1016/S1743-9191(06)60023-X.
8. Anderson RR, Parrish JA. Selective photothermolysis: precise microsurgery by selective absorption of pulsed radiation. Science. 1983;220(4596):524–27. https://doi.org/10.1126/science.6836297.
9. Shokrollahi K, Raymond E, Murison MSC. Lasers: principles and surgical applications. The Journal of Surgery. 2014;28–34. https://doi.org/10.1016/S1743-9191(06)60023-X.

10. Shokrollahi K. The laser test patch. Ann Plast Surg. 2016;77:373–5.
11. Nehal KS, Levine VJ, Ross B, Ashinoff R. Comparison of high-energy pulsed carbon dioxide laser resurfacing and dermabrasion in the revision of surgical scars. Dermatol Surg. 1998;24:647–50.
12. Becker DW. Use of the carbon dioxide laser in treating multiple cutaneous neurofibromas. Ann Plast Surg. 1991;26:582–6.
13. Kilmer SL, Lee MS, Grevelink JM, Flotte TJ, Anderson RR. The Q-switched Nd:YAG laser effectively treats tattoos. A controlled, dose-response study. Arch Dermatol. 1993;129:971–8.
14. Tan OT, Murray S, Kurban AK. Action spectrum of vascular specific injury using pulsed irradiation. J Invest Dermatol. 1989;92:868–71.
15. Edström DW, Ros AM. The treatment of port-wine stains with the pulsed dye laser at 600 nm. Br J Dermatol. 1997;136:360–3.
16. Al-Mohamady AE, Ibrahim SM, Muhammad MM. Pulsed dye laser versus long-pulsed Nd:YAG laser in the treatment of hypertrophic scars and keloid: a comparative randomized split-scar trial. J Cosmet Laser Ther. 2016;8:1–5.
17. Koike S, Akaishi S, Nagashima Y, Dohi T, Hyakusoku H, Ogawa R. Nd:YAG laser treatment for keloids and hypertrophic scars: an analysis of 102 cases. Plast Reconstr Surg Glob Open. 2015;2(12):e272.

Carbon Dioxide Laser Treatment for Scars

Swati Kannan and David Ozog

1 Introduction

Scar formation occurs as a common end point of skin injury penetrating the basement membrane or as a result of prolonged inflammatory conditions. Scars tend to be less compliant than healthy skin and lack cutaneous appendages such as hair follicles, sebaceous glands, and apocrine or eccrine sweat glands [1]. Even though most scars do not pose health risks, some scars cause significant disfigurement, pruritus, pain, and functional impairment [2].

Proper classification of scars is necessary for appropriate treatment as differences in scar color, texture, and morphology affect laser type and parameters [3]. The main classification categories consist of normotrophic, hypertrophic, keloidal, and atrophic scars. [3, 4] Hypertrophic scars result from uncontrolled proliferation of fibroblasts and excess formation of extracellular matrix (ECM) forming raised, firm erythematous scars confined to the boundaries of initial skin injury [3, 5]. The formation of keloids is similar to hypertrophic scars but the collagen bundles cross the limits of the original wound and do not regress over time. Atrophic scars appear as depressions caused by collagen destruction and often occur after inflammatory processes such as cystic acne.

Various therapies have been advocated for different scar types including intralesional corticosteroid injections, bleomycin, 5-fluorouracil, silicone gel sheeting, chemical peels, radiation, cryosurgery, surgical excision, as well as several laser and light devices [2, 6, 7]. Nonetheless, treatment of cutaneous scars remains a challenge due to a lack of randomized controlled trials and unsatisfactory outcomes.

In the past 30 years, introduction of laser technology and multiple refinements in treatment parameters have placed laser devices at the forefront of scar therapy. Laser skin resurfacing of atrophic acne scars is one of the earliest treatments performed with ablative lasers such as the carbon dioxide (CO_2) laser and the erbium-doped yttrium-aluminum-garnet (Er:YAG) [8]. These lasers emit high-energy, short pulse duration impulses that vaporize intra- and extracellular water, causing tissue ablation with limited thermal conduction to surrounding tissue. Since energy is limited to nontargeted tissues, the likelihood of additional scarring is reduced [9]. Despite its effectiveness in scar revision, continuous wave laser ablation can cause undesirable cutaneous side effects such as hypertrophic scarring and prolonged erythema [8].

The increased risks with continuous ablation steered the development of fractional photothermolysis, which has revolutionized laser scar surgery. Fractional ablative CO_2 lasers (10,600 nm) create microscopic columns or thermal wounds of variable depths into the skin. These channels are surrounded by normal skin, referred to as microthermal zones (MTZ) (see Figure 1). The pixilated pattern of holes enables tensionless neocollagenesis within the MTZs, leading to dermal remodeling and faster healing times compared to continuous wave ablation [7]. When treating patients, it is important to remember that the "fraction" of skin treated is inversely proportional to the depth created with these devices. Superficial treatment of 20–50 microns (μm) in depth at 80–100% surface density will have much different biochemical effects than deep treatment at 1000 μm and 5% surface density.

After fractional photothermolysis, the treated skin demonstrates conversion to a fetal collagen profile with an increase in collagen III deposition and diminished collagen type I bundles, elevated heat shock proteins and smooth muscle [10–12]. The rehabilitated tissue reveals normal collagen architecture and vasculature allowing for improvement in texture and erythema [13]. Even though scars show decreased clinical erythema after fractional CO_2 laser therapy, CD31 analysis indicates a paradoxical increase in the density of normal blood vessels [14]. This immunohistochemical finding contradicts prior notions that clinical erythema is

S. Kannan, MD (✉)
Department of Dermatology, Kaiser Southern California Permanente Medical Group, Riverside, CA, USA

D. Ozog, MD
Department of Dermatology, Henry Ford Hospital, Detroit, MI, USA
e-mail: dozog1@hfhs.org

K. Shokrollahi (ed.), *Laser Management of Scars*, https://doi.org/10.1007/978-3-030-52919-2_5

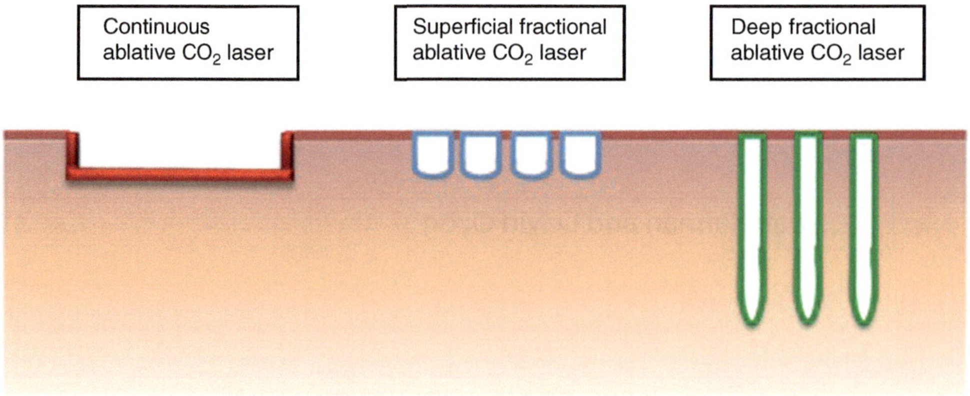

Fig. 1 The diagram depicts the difference between a traditional CO_2 laser, which ablates the epithelium and underlying superficial dermis in a continuous fashion. The fractional system creates microscopic channels into the dermis, surrounded by normal tissue, referred to as the microthermal zone (MTZ). The superficial settings create shallow channels whereas the deep fractional CO_2 laser produces deeper channels into the dermis at much lower surface densities

mainly caused by dilated vasculature. Improvements in clinical erythema are due to multifactorial causes with both density and distribution of vasculature and underlying collagen architecture playing major roles [13].

As explained above, the various properties of fractional CO_2 lasers are being exploited for treatment of atrophic scars, traumatic, and postsurgical scars. This chapter will focus on the treatment and prevention of various scar types with both fractional and ablative CO_2 lasers.

2 Review of the Evidence

2.1 Hypertrophic Scars Including Burn and Surgical Scars

Hypertrophic scars develop from overzealous expression of collagen and appear as firm, red and raised plaques. They more likely exhibit symptoms of pruritus or tenderness compared to their atrophic counterparts. For treatment of these scars, consistent evidence points to the effectiveness of pulsed dye laser (PDL, 585/595 nm) and non-ablative fractional lasers in improving scar erythema, pliability, and thickness [2, 3, 15]. In 1980s, a few studies investigated continuous wave CO_2 ablation for excision or debulking of hypertrophic scars and keloids with contradictory results [16, 17]. Due to recurrence of these scars and unwanted side effects, focus was then diverted to non-ablative systems such as the PDL laser. In 1998, years prior to the now ubiquitous fractional devices, Alster et al. performed one of the first split-scar studies of hypertrophic scars in 20 patients, examining the effects of CO_2 vaporization alone compared to a combination of CO_2 and PDL treatment. This study demonstrated significant textural and clinical improvement in dually treated scars compared to CO_2 de-epithelialization alone [18]. The challenge with fully ablative devices was that the thermal injury had the potential to worsen the scar, and these devices were relegated to "debulking" rather than scar treatment or rehabilitation. Since that time, PDL has been considered as the gold standard of laser treatment for erythematous hypertrophic scars.

After the advent of the fractional CO_2 laser, other investigations evaluated the effectiveness of fractional photothermolysis on hypertrophic scars and keloids, including burn scars. Compared to keloids and hypertrophic scars, thermal burn scars can be more disfiguring and are often associated with physical and psychological disabilities. Third-degree burns are characterized by altered texture, pliability, and elasticity that all worsen with time [8]. Interestingly, over time many burn patients complain about this altered "feel" of their skin more than the accompanying disfigurement. In 2008, Haedersal reported the first burn scar treated successfully with a fractional CO_2 laser after a single-pass using two different settings: medium and high-density coverage. Three months after just one treatment, skin texture and color improved using the high-density pass [19]. Similarly, Waibel and Beer demonstrated enhanced texture and appearance of a third-degree burn scar after a single treatment of ablative fractional CO_2 laser with two passes [20].

Much of the authors' research has focused on histopathological analysis of burn scars after treatment with fractional CO_2 laser to assess molecular basis for improvement. Revised scars exhibited regression to a fetal collagen profile with increased collagen type III and decreased collagen type I, leading to clinical improvement [10]. Treated burn scars also demonstrated upregulation of matrix metalloproteinase-1 (MMP-1), which contributes to collagen (scar) breakdown prior to remodeling [21]. Since these preliminary studies, an increasing body of literature has developed, supporting the use of fractional ablative lasers for burn/hypertrophic scar rehabilitation. In fact, a recent consensus report on laser treatment of hypertrophic traumatic scars recommends the use of ablative fractional lasers over all others for robust collagen remodeling required within the deeper dermis. For device selection, the authors suggest fractional CO_2 devices as these lasers tend to coagulate the surrounding tissue more so than erbium:YAG lasers [22].

More recent investigations by our group, and supported by Azzam et al. and El-Zawahry, illustrated improvement in scar scores after treatment of hypertrophic scars with fractional CO_2 laser; however, keloids proved resistant to clinical improvement. Since most CO_2 lasers only penetrate about 400–1000 μm into the dermis, thicker keloids, and hypertrophic scars at certain laser energies may not be as responsive as superficial scars [4, 23]. These studies mainly noted enhanced pliability in both scar types, but the effects on vascularity, scar height, and dyspigmentation were less pronounced. Even though histopathologic analysis revealed collagen remodeling with parallel arrangement of collagen and a decrease in collagen density in all patients, clinically the improvements were not significant.

However, some devices can penetrate significantly deeper and may have novel effects on thicker scars. An Italian study of 50 consecutive patients with mature keloids treated with a high-energy pulsed CO_2 laser and subsequent topical hyaluronic acid application demonstrated reduction in scar height and texture after four treatments [24]. The authors have had moderate success with truncal keloids treated with deep fractional CO_2 at a depth of 1000+ μm and low densities of 3–5%, followed by immediate application of triamcinolone acetonide 40 mg/cc. The fenestration with the laser allows the steroid to diffuse evenly throughout the keloid.

2.2 Atrophic Scars

Atrophic scars appear as dermal depressions caused by collagen destruction after inflammatory skin diseases such as cystic acne or varicella; occasionally, this form of scar occurs after trauma or surgery. Therapies such as chemical peels, surgical excision, punch grafting, dermabrasion, and soft-tissue augmentation using dermal fillers have been attempted with varying levels of success. Prior to the advent of fractional devices, ablative CO_2 resurfacing of atrophic acne scars showed 50–80% improvement. However, this improvement was attributed to laser ablation of adjacent tissue rather than augmentation of the atrophic tissue. Even though this resulted in an improved clinical and cosmetic appearance, normal tissue was not increased in atrophic areas. Additionally, fully ablative treatments were not without risks and significant side effects [3, 9]. Patients experienced post-treatment erythema lasting for weeks to months, edema, burning sensation, milia, exacerbation of acne, crusting, and intermittent pruritus. Other noteworthy complications such as infection, scarring, alterations in skin texture, post-inflammatory hyperpigmentation in darker skin types, delayed-onset hypopigmentation, and increased probability of contact dermatitis to topical preparations can also occur as a result of continuous tissue ablation [9, 25, 26].

Due to the aforementioned risks and different treatment goals and parameters, recent evidence points to fractional CO_2 laser as being an effective ablative device for revision of atrophic scars, especially acne scars [2, 7, 9]. Additionally, a comparison between the fractional and fully ablative CO_2 lasers proves that the fractional laser improves scar appearance more so than the ablative system. In a study of 60 patients with atrophic scars secondary to cutaneous leishmaniasis, fractional CO_2 laser treatment showed 76.7% improvement at the 6-month interval versus 44.7% in the ablative CO_2 laser group [27]. These results are concordant with other studies that also demonstrate patient improvement scores of 26–50% for non-acne atrophic scars with a fractional laser [28].

Topographic analysis in 13 patients with acne scars demonstrated an average of 67% improvement after 2–3 treatments with fractional CO_2 laser; a higher degree of improvement correlated with higher energy levels of 70–100 mJ [9]. As there are various morphologies of acne scars, not all respond well to CO_2 laser treatments. A study of 60 patients (skin types II–IV) with acne scars of various types illustrated that fractional CO_2 laser improved rolling and superficial boxcar scars significantly, but pitted/ice pick-type scars responded the least to laser monotherapy. In fact, the 11 patients with >75% improvement in their scars had mainly rolling scars. This observation carries therapeutic weight as patients with predominantly ice pick or pitted scars receive supplementary treatment with chemical reconstruction by 80–100% trichloroacetic acid (TCA CROSS technique) in the authors' clinics [29]. In darker skin types, post-inflammatory hyperpigmentation can also occur, which ensued in three out of the 60 patients in this study group [30]. However, this does not need to be a limiting factor in treating patients with skin types III–VI, since this acute hyperpigmentation reliably fades over time as opposed to chronic hyperpigmentation from inflammatory conditions. Prior to performing laser treatment for darker skin types, the authors discuss the risks of hyperpigmentation with these patients and explain that the discoloration is technically not a "scar" and will fade over time (weeks to months) as the depressed areas improve.

Laser monotherapy is not always maximally effective for atrophic scars, as dermal fillers may be needed to augment the depressed tissue. In this case, the creation of microscopic noncontiguous columns by fractional lasers can be used to deliver larger molecules into the deeper dermis without injections. The combination of ablative fractional laser and topical poly-L-lactic acid (PLLA, Sculptra®) may synergistically up-regulate collagen synthesis. In a study of 19 patients with atrophic scars from various injuries, ablative fractional CO_2 laser followed by application of PLLA improved scar atrophy, dyschromia/color mismatch, and contour by at least 33% (in each criteria) [7]. Similarly, as stated previously, fractional CO_2 laser combined with application of topical steroids has been demonstrated to augment hypertrophic scar treatment [31]. Thus, fractional CO_2 laser–assisted drug delivery of a topical steroid (hypertrophic scar or keloid) or PLLA (atrophic scar) can further modify the landscape of scar treatments [32].

While most investigations substantiate that ablative fractional photothermolysis improve atrophic scars, Vandrooge and colleagues demonstrate no improvement in either atrophic or hypertrophic scars after fractional CO_2 laser treatment. The authors hypothesize this could be due to several factors—scar location, scar type, and scar age. Facial atrophic scars may respond more readily to fractional CO_2 revision compared to other scar types on the body [33].

2.3 Contracted Scars/Range of Motion

One of the most exciting advances in scar treatment is the ability of deep fractional CO_2 lasers to improve functional deficits caused by scar contractures. Shumaker et al. demonstrated improvement in function and range of motion in four patients with scar contractures located on the extremities and trunk. Patients were treated with pulse energies ranging from 17.5 to 50 mJ to obtain depths up to 2 mm with densities ranging from 5 to 15%. This case series was one of the first investigations highlighting the effectiveness of low-density deep fractional lasers for the treatment of scar contractures caused by a variety of injuries. [34] A low density of 5% indicates that within a 1-cm treatment area, 95% of the area is left unablated. However, the actual "treatment" area is greater since there is a thermal zone around each ablated area which undergoes remodeling. At higher energy levels, lower densities are needed to prevent additional scarring or burns.

Similar results occurred in pediatric patients with scar contractures of their hands secondary to third-degree burns and in cases of severe contractures related to split-thickness skin grafts on the forearms [35, 36]. In this study, Krakowski et al. demonstrated functional improvement even after a single treatment with deep fractional CO_2 laser at low-density settings of 3–5%. The authors have produced consistent results in clinic, with functional improvements of morphea-related contractures, postsurgical contractures, traumatic injuries, and burn scars. In addition to the low-density deep CO_2 settings for improvement in range of motion, the authors treat these scars with a superficial depth and higher density to obtain improvements in hyperpigmentation and skin texture [10]. As seen in Fig. 2, after three treatments with low-density deep fractional and high-density superficial fractional CO_2, significant improvements in texture, discoloration, and contraction were noted in this patient with a contracted scar caused by morphea on the left posterior thigh. Reduction in pain and improvement in range of motion with participation in collegiate athletics were also seen. Previously, she had minimal benefit with over 157 treatments with ultraviolet A (UVA1) therapy.

Enhancement in both range of motion and wound healing of chronic ulcers can be perceived with treatment of surrounding hypertrophic scars with fractional photothermolysis. Treatment of these contracted areas reduces tension adjacent to the chronic ulcer, thus releasing the contraction and inducing rapid wound healing via secondary intention. The authors treated a patient, who suffered from an axillary scar contracture after CO_2 excision of extensive hidradenitis suppurativa lesions, with high-energy, low-density CO_2 treatments. Due to tension caused by surrounding hypertrophic scar tissue, she had open non-

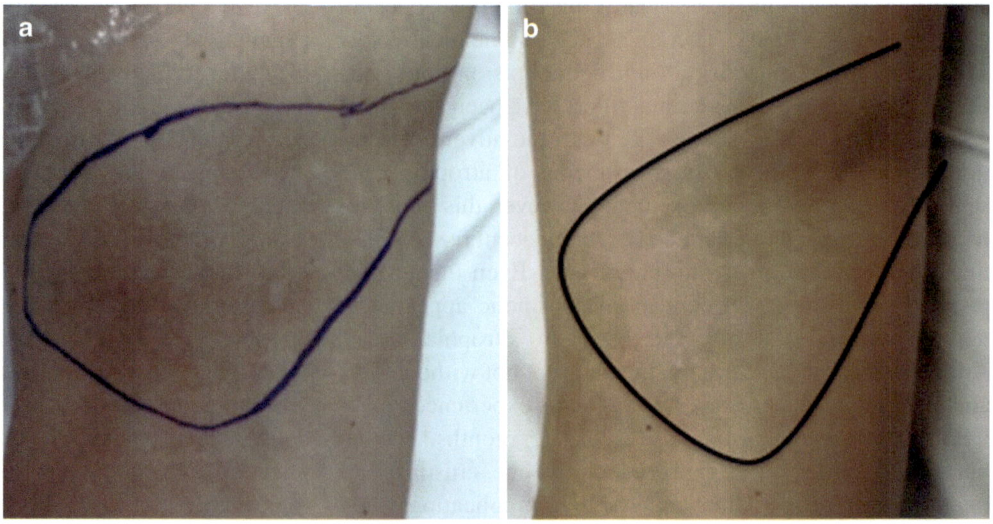

Fig. 2 (**a**) This picture shows a hyperpigmented contracted plaque secondary to morphea on the left posterior thigh. (**b**) After three treatments with deep fractional CO2 at low densities of 3–5% and energy of 50 mJ, and superficial active CO_2 at higher energies of 80–100 mJ, one can note improvements in hyperpigmentation and induration of the scar. Patient had a total of five treatments, resulting in significant decrease in pain and scar contracture and recovery of range of motion and function

healing ulcerations within the axilla that persisted after several months. Treatment with four sessions at low-density settings healed the erosions completely and improved the axillary range of motion significantly [37]. The results shown in our clinics are consistent with other studies. For instance, Shumaker et al. described a case series of three patients with chronic wounds secondary to explosive injuries; wound healing was observed within a few weeks of the first treatment with fractional CO_2 laser at high energies and low densities [38]. Treatment of these wounds with fractional photothermolysis is comparable to dermabrasion, but the creation of microcolumns provides advantages over dermabrasion as normal tissue is present for collagen remodeling. Additionally, the laser most likely disrupts the bacterial biofilms and destroys dysfunctional scar tissue, which both potentiate the chronicity of non-healing wounds [38]. Reepithelialized wounds after fractional resurfacing tend to remain epithelialized several months after treatment, as shown in two pediatric cases with chronic wounds [39]. However, more investigations are needed to validate the efficacy of fractional laser treated chronic ulcerations, as the abovementioned evidence is based on anecdotes or small case series.

3 Early Treatment/Scar Prevention

Many of these studies focus on revision of established older scars, but evidence suggests that early physical treatment or intraoperative treatment can affect and improve the final trajectory of surgical scars. The concept of early intervention for scar reduction was demonstrated by a preliminary non-laser study prior to the myriad of laser treatments. In this report, dermabrasion of full-thickness edges during wound closure resulted in no visible scar in darker phenotypes [40]. The rationale behind early postoperative laser intervention is to influence the fibroblasts and myofibroblasts that migrate into the wound base within the first week after injury. An abraded superficial wound exhibits different biochemical properties favoring scarless healing, compared to a deeper incisional wound. This concept was tested in a split-scar, blinded observer study performed by Ozog, D and Moy, R. Intraoperative treatment of the suture line with superficial depth, high surface density fractional CO_2 laser resulted in dramatic improvement of the final cosmetic appearance of surgical repairs [41]. The effectiveness of early intervention using fractional photothermolysis has also been demonstrated in post-thyroidectomy scars [42]. Following those initial studies, Lee et al. performed a split-scar study of various scar locations in 15 patients, with the first treatment at 3 weeks postoperatively utilizing a fractional CO_2 laser. Three months after the second treatment, the treated side demonstrated statistically significant reduction in Vancouver Scar Scale (VSS) scores compared to the controls. There was notable improvement in scar texture and thickness [43]. The same results do not occur with low surface density and high-depth settings. In a study of 20 patients, half of the surgical scars were treated at suture removal with deep fractional CO_2 laser at low surface density. However, the VSS scores failed to detect a significant difference between the treated and untreated sides 3 months after one treatment. A statistical reduction was only seen with the patient visual analog scores (VAS), signifying the patients preferred the treated site over the control. Perhaps, patients could detect an improvement in the deeper non-visible portion of the scar [44]. In either case, early treatment with a fractional device is safe based on these studies. The main side effects of fractional laser reported in these studies included pain during the procedure and posttreatment edema, erythema, and scaling which resolved within 1 week. Hyperpigmentation has also been reported which resolves over weeks to months [28, 44]. Early treatment may favorably alter the ultimate trajectory of scar formation and should be considered in all appropriate surgical repairs, particularly in cosmetically sensitive areas.

4 Treatment Methodology

Prior to beginning scar treatments with ablative devices, the following elements should be considered:

1. During the initial evaluation, patient history should include the following pertinent aspects: prior history of herpes simplex virus (for peri-oral treatments), prior surgeries performed and scar history (tendency to form hypertrophic or keloidal scars), past and current medical conditions, history of radiation, and current medications including herbal products and drug allergies.
2. Physical examination should document the following: skin type, evidence of photodamage, scar characteristics such as erythema, pliability, textural irregularity, dyspigmentation, scar thickness, and any presence of scar contractures.
3. A high-quality photograph emphasizing the scar and topography of the treatment area should be obtained prior to onset of treatments and at each follow-up visit [45]. A particularly helpful technique is to use oblique/side lighting to create shadows within and around the scars. This highlights scar depressions and elevations. Front flash should be avoided as this mutes the true clinical picture by minimizing shadows. If a camera with a side-mounted flash is being used, simply cover one flash, then the other.
4. As with any dermatologic procedure, the physician should conduct a thorough discussion with the patient, including realistic expectations, therapeutic goals, and potential

Table 1 This table lists the side effects that commonly occur with ablative fractional resurfacing of large areas (AFR)

Common complications	Rarer complications
Procedural pain	Infection
Transient erythema/ localized edema	Prolonged erythema (>1 month posttreatment with AFR)
Pinpoint bleeding (reflects depth into papillary dermis/may be desirable in some scar types)	Transient post-inflammatory hyperpigmentation or hypopigmentation (which takes longer to resolve in darker skin types)
Mild serous drainage/ crusting for 24–48 h	Scarring–particularly, hypertrophic scarring (especially with treatment of the neck/inadequate cooling) [48, 49]
Mild post-procedural pain (relieved by cold ice packs or mild oral analgesics)	Post-procedural pain requiring oral narcotics
Delayed purpura/ ecchymoses	Anesthesia toxicity
Acne, milia (occurs more so with resurfacing and less with localized treatment)	Ectropion formation (over treatment of lower eyelid)

These side effects should be discussed, even in smaller treatment areas [48–50].

complications (see Table 1). Subsequently, a written consent should be signed by both the patient and physician.

5. If the patient has a history of herpes labialis, and the procedure is to be performed on the face, viral prophylaxis is recommended. However, some physicians prescribe preoperative antivirals and antibiotics to all patients [46].
6. The majority of the laser scar treatments with ablative or fractional CO_2 laser occurs in a clinical office setting. For low density and superficial settings, it is often possible to use cold air/ice for anesthesia, which minimizes patient time and potential discomfort of injections. Patients can apply commercially available topical anesthetic preparations such as Eutectic Mixture of Local Anesthesia (EMLA) 60 min prior to the procedure. An hour or longer is recommended for topical anesthesia application as the continuous and fractional ablative CO_2 laser exert their action in the deeper dermis. It is important to avoid topical anesthesia on inflamed areas or denuded skin. Additionally, for larger treatment areas, product application should be limited to the most sensitive areas ("hot spots") [47]. Smaller areas can often be injected with local anesthetics and are well tolerated.
7. Prior to laser treatment, topical anesthetics are completely removed to avoid any impediment to laser–tissue interactions. Patient comfort during scar revision can be augmented with the use of a cooling device. Despite these measures, local anesthesia, regional nerve blockade with infiltrative anesthesia, and oral benzodiazepine may be necessary for pain relief if large areas are being treated with deeper settings [47].
8. Lastly, ensure proper eye protection is in place for the patient, the physician, and any assistant in the room.

5 General Instructions for Laser Operation

1. Hold the hand piece perpendicularly to the lesion as the treatment area is traversed.
2. Ensure a cooling device precedes the laser firing to adequately cool the treatment area if not an integrated device.
3. Wipe the char from the treated areas with wet gauze, as dry gauze is flammable.

6 Laser Specifications

Although fully ablative and fractional CO_2 lasers differ in certain technical aspects, particular characteristics are similar between devices. All CO_2 lasers carry a wavelength of 10,600 nm in the infrared range, which specifically targets the chromophore water. In order to ablate the target without disproportionate surrounding thermal damage, it is preferred to deliver a minimum fluence of 5 J/cm^2 with a pulse duration of <1 millisecond (ms), characterized as the thermal relaxation time of skin [50].

Multiple fractional CO_2 devices are currently available on the market. Even though basic principles apply to these lasers, specific settings differ per machine. Thus, users should familiarize themselves with the depth and surface area coverage correlating with the various parameters of energy, power, and density pertaining to the device. Please refer to Table 2 for general comparison between the available manufacturers.

This section will focus on the specifications of the Lumenis UltraPulse® fractional CO_2 laser for scar treatment, as the authors use this device. Separate handpieces, Active Fx, and Deep Fx, deliver ablation at various depths. The Active Fx handpiece, with a spot size of 1.3 mm is used for superficial skin treatments. It delivers energy from 2 mJ (150 mJ/cm^2) to 225 mJ (169 J/cm^2) with power settings from 1 W (4.4 Hz) to 60 W (600 Hz); 70 mJ pertains to a depth of 40 μm, and 225 mJ reaches a depth of 242 μm. In general, using the Active Fx handpiece, superficial ablative wounds extending into the upper papillary dermis can be created with one to two passes [31, 51]. When performing two passes, the char from the first pass is often removed with moist gauze. The most common indications for multiple passes in the same session are peri-oral rhytids and cheek rhytids, which often have a thicker dermal component.

The Deep Fx handpiece offers two treatment modes: Deep Fx and SCAAR Fx. The former mode is utilized for treating more profound rhytids, acne scars, and other deep cosmetic scars, whereas the SCAAR Fx produces a greater impact for

Table 2 This is a list of some CO_2 laser devices that are currently available on the market, at the time of authorship. This list is not complete, and there might be other devices on the market by date of publication

Manufacturer	Delivery mode	Spot size	Pulse duration (ms)	Depth	Energy per treatment spot (mJ)	Average power/peak power	Overall scanned area
Alma lasers-Pixel CO2		50 mm/100 mm	0.05–1.0			70 W (peak)	7 × 7 mm; 9 × 9 mm
DEKA SmartXide [2]	Scanned conventional	0.35 mm	0.2–2.0	500–800 μm	<50	40,60,80 W/250 W	15 × 15 mm
Ellipse Juvia	Scanned	0.5 mm	0.2–7.0	100–400 μm	10–20	15 W (peak)	7 × 7 mm; 9 × 9 mm; 11 × 11 mm
Lasering USA MiXto SX	Scanned (four quadrant)	300 μm/180 μm (second gen)	2.5–16	Ablation 100–150 or 300–500 μm	20–30	30 W (peak)	20 × 20 mm
Lutronic eCO2 plus	Static and dynamic	0.12 mm	0.3–0.6	400–600 μm	10–20	40 W/60 W	12 × 12 mm
Reliant repair	Paintbrush continous motion	135 μm	0.15–3.0	650–1600 μm	10–20	N/A	15 mm × 4 cm
Syneron CO2RE	Articulated arm	0.15 mm	0.02–3	20–750 μm	<90	30 W/60 W	10 × 10 mm
UltraPulse Lumenis – Active Fx – Deep Fx	Scanned pattern generator	–1.3 mm –0.12 mm	<1	–10–300 μm –150–1600 μm	–2–225 –2.5–50	60 W/240 W	10 × 10 mm

Table 3 Energy settings and surface area coverage per treatment location

	Active Fx energy settings (mJ)	Coverage density (for Active Fx)[a]	Deep Fx energy settings (mJ)	Coverage density (for deep Fx)
Facial skin	>100–125	73–95%[b]	15–22.5	5–15%
Periorbital skin	60–90	73–80%	8–10	5–15%
Peri-oral skin	90–125	73–95%[b]	15–22.5	5–15%
Neck/chest/ extremities	70–80	55–68%	8–10	5–15%
Hypertrophic scar	80–125	68–100%	12.5–20	10–15%
Contracted burn scars	80–100	68–100%	17.5–50	5–15%[a]
Acne scars (face)	80–125	80–100%	20–30	10–15%
Scar prevention	80–125	68%	No evidence	No evidence

These are just guidelines as treatment parameters should be customized to patient skin type, scar type, pain tolerance, and location. The authors often use settings based on prior patient experience and response to the laser device during therapy.
[a]The density coverage should decrease as pulse energies increase for treatment of contracted scars with deep fractional CO_2.
[b]May perform second pass for deeper rhytids [10, 33, 34, 36, 41, 44, 51, 52].

thick complex lesions, creating a depth up to 4 mm with a single pulse. The Deep Fx offers a spot size of 0.12 mm, energy settings between 2.5 and 50 mJ, which corresponds to a tissue depth of 75–1500 μm, respectively. Alternatively, SCAAR Fx produces energy settings of 10–150 mJ, reaching depths of 300 and 3200 μm, respectively. The density can be altered with the fractional CO_2 lasers, unlike the traditional ablative devices. Based on the density used, partial or full ablation can be achieved with the superficial Active Fx [51]. See Table 3 for energy and density ranges depending on treatment location and scar type. Typically, the authors perform the deep ablation first without skip or overlap areas, laying scanned imprints adjacent to one another. If necessary, superficial treatment with Active Fx is subsequently performed with 10% overlap between laser beams to allow maximum coverage of treatment area. Feathering is often performed at treatment edges to minimize any potential geographic erythema corresponding to the shape used. This is performed by keeping the handpiece in motion while delivering the laser pulse.

In general, for hypertrophic scars, higher fluences and densities are required for deeper penetration of energy. A preferred setting for Deep Fx mode may depend on the observation of pinpoint bleeding upon treatment. Pinpoint bleeding indicates penetration into the papillary dermis. For most scars, authors start at lower energy and density settings and customize the parameters based on the patient's tolerance of pain, skin type, and scar type. To enhance treatment results for hypertrophic scars or atrophic scars, subsequent triamcinolone acetonide injectable suspension (Kenalog®) and filler (hyaluronic acid or PLLA) can be applied, respectively [31].

Postoperative care with cold vinegar soaks and dressings with petrolatum will minimize adverse events and accelerate healing. Application of petrolatum-based ointment should be continued several times daily until the treated site is fully epithelialized. Photo-protection with sun avoidance in early post-treatment period and bland sunblocks should also be utilized [52]. Various studies also demonstrate faster healing rates after laser abrasion using occlusive silicone-based dressings and topical vitamin C [53, 54]. In fact, a recently published study illustrated that postoperative delivery of Vitamin C, E, and Ferulic acid decreased edema and erythema within the first week of treatment [55].

Low-level laser therapy, such as a light-emitting diode (LED, 590 nm), has also been used to decrease post-treatment erythema. Studies by Weiss and colleagues showed decreased erythema and improved efficacy of laser rejuvenation with the accompaniment of LED photomodulation [56]. Alster corroborated these findings by treating 20 patients with LED photomodulation after full-face fractional resurfacing. The LED- treated facial halves demonstrated decreased erythema at 24, 48, and 96 hours after treatment [57].

7 Clinical Examples

The examples listed in this section include a combination of treatment modalities for optimal scar revision and patient satisfaction. These procedures were performed in the authors' specialty "scar clinic" by dermatology residents, under the supervision of an attending procedural dermatologist. Prior to each procedure, photos were taken of the scar or treatment area, and the Vancouver Scar Scale (VSS) was used to grade the scar. This is a commonly used scar assessment scale, with a potential score ranging from 0 (no scar) to 13 (most severe scar). Most patients had one to three treatments performed every 6–12 weeks.

7.1 Case #1

A 60-year-old Caucasian female presented 3 months after Mohs surgery of a basal cell carcinoma and subsequent primary closure located on the left lower eyelid. The resulting scar appeared as a pink, linear, contracted scar. No ectropion of the left eye was seen but the scar was tethering the fine thin infraorbital skin (Fig. 3). The VSS prior to any treatments was eight out of 13. Patient underwent one laser treatment with potassium titanyl phosphate (KTP) device to treat the erythema and two fractional CO_2 laser treatments using both the Active Fx and Deep Fx modalities, at 3-month intervals. The settings for Active Fx remained consistent for both treatments at energy of 80 millijoules (mJ) and a density of 5 (surface coverage of ~100%). The Deep Fx delivered a range of 20–40 mJ at a coverage of 10%; settings were calibrated at each visit based on scar texture, pigmentation, and observation of pinpoint bleeding. VSS score decreased to a score of one after two treatments with improvement in contraction, vasculature, and overall cosmetic appearance of the scar.

7.2 Case #2

A 32-year-old Caucasian female presented with a deeply atrophic scar on the left shoulder caused by morphea profundus. The scar had been present for 8 months as she had inactive disease after oral methotrexate treatment. Physical examination revealed a 3 × 1 cm, deeply atrophic, indurated, and slightly hyperpigmented scar with dilated telangiectasias along the scar base. Scar revision included three treatments of KTP, 532 nm, laser and five treatments of both superficial and deep modalities of fractional CO_2 laser followed by topical PLLA application and injection. VSS score decreased from 7/13 to 3/13 after five treatments (Table 4). Even though the atrophic component improved significantly, patient developed mild hypertrophic scarring centrally; nonetheless, patient was satisfied with the results, as the large depression had resolved (Fig. 4).

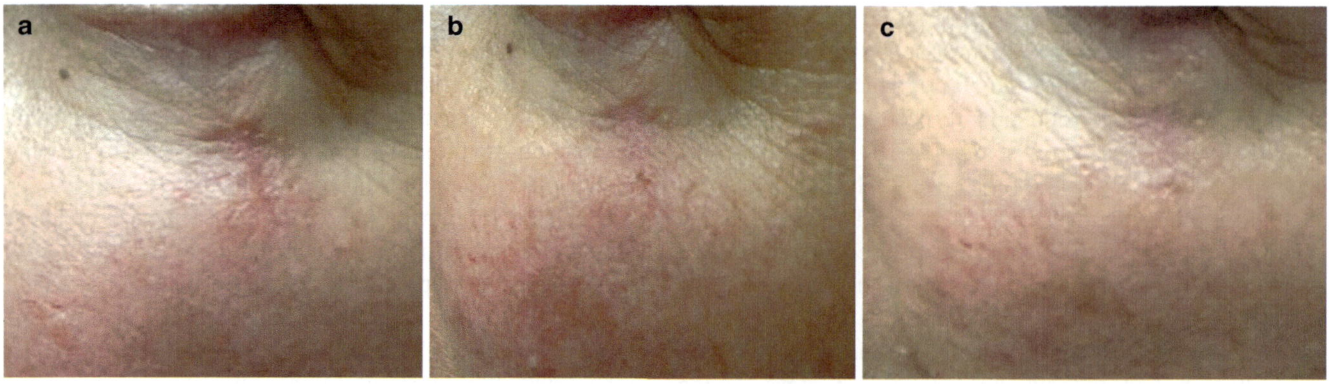

Fig. 3 (**a**) Prior to any treatments, a pink contracted linear scar is visible. (**b**) Three months after the first treatment, a significant decrease in scar contraction is noted. (**c**) After two treatments, normalization of the scar and decreased erythema are both observed

Table 4 Treatment settings for fractional CO_2 Active and Deep Fx are listed as energy/density

	Treatment 1	Treatment 2	Treatment 3	Treatment 4	Treatment 5
Active Fx	N/A	80 mJ/5	80 mJ/5	80 mJ/5	80 mJ/5
Deep Fx	15 mJ/15	50 mJ/5	50 mJ/10	50 mJ/10	50 mJ/10
KTP	10/10/8	10/10/8	10/10/9	N/A	N/A

Settings for KTP are formatted as spot size in millimeters (mm)/pulse duration in milliseconds (ms)/fluence in Joules per area squared (J/cm^2)

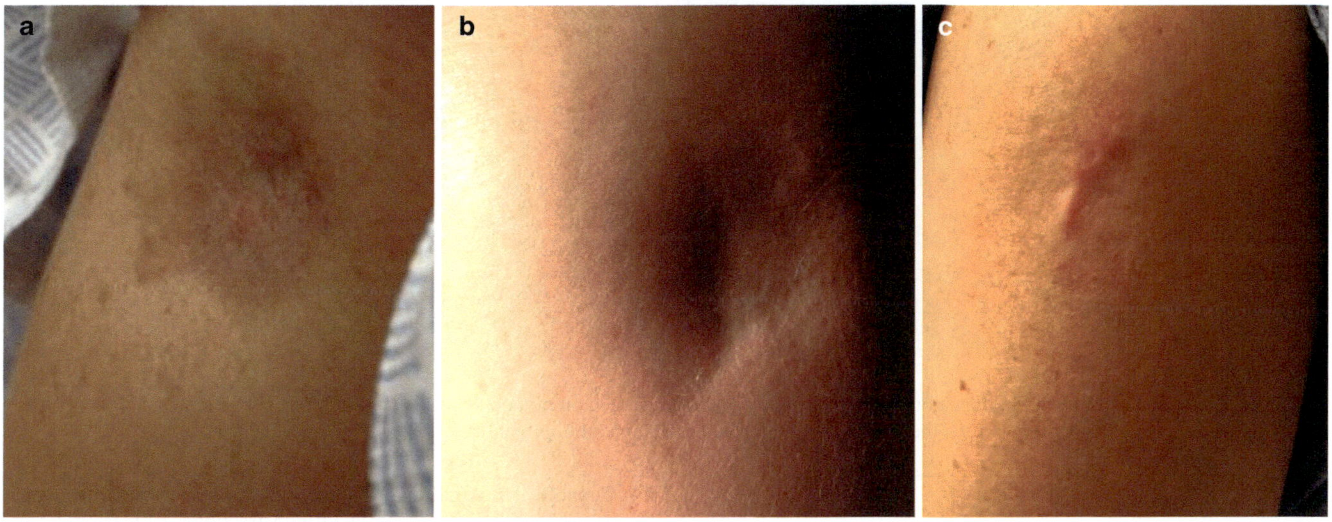

Fig. 4 (**a**) Prior to any treatments, a deeply atrophic, mildly hyperpigmented, indurated plaque with prominent vasculature was observed. (**b**) After two treatments, no significant difference was observed in the atrophic component but the violaceous and hyperpigmented discoloration improved. (**c**) After five treatments, the atrophic component fully resolved with normal resilience of skin texture; however, a resulting hypertrophic scar formed, which is a reported complication of CO_2 laser treatment

7.3 Case #3

A 17-year-old Caucasian male with acne scarring on bilateral cheeks and temples for 3 years presented for facial resurfacing. Patient underwent one treatment of KTP and two treatments of fractional CO_2 laser with subsequent topical application of PLLA. The first CO_2 treatment was conducted using only the Deep Fx handpiece, at an energy level of 15 mJ and density of 15. The second treatment included Active Fx at an energy setting of 80 mJ and density at 3 and Deep Fx at 17.5 mJ and density of 20. Even though the VSS scores did not change, patient noted significant improvement of erythema and skin texture after just two treatments (Fig. 5). Unfortunately after the second treatment, patient was lost to follow-up.

8 Discussion

Fractional laser devices treat scars with fewer side effects and less downtime than traditionally ablative CO_2 lasers, thus favoring fractional devices for scar revision and skin resurfacing. By leaving uninjured tissue around each microscopic channel or thermal zone, the intact dermis heals faster around these columns, stimulating gradual collagen remodeling [58].

A large body of literature now supports fractional ablative CO_2 laser treatment to successfully revise scars, especially atrophic scars. Additional work supports the unique ability of these devices to improve function and range of motion with restrictive scars. Most studies focus on mature scars, which have been present for months to years after surgery or trauma. However, more recent investigations demonstrate effectiveness of early scar revision with these devices, performed within the first few weeks of surgery [41–44].

For optimal cosmetic and functional results, different modalities of treatments can be combined to provide synergistic effects. An example includes dual treatment with a vascular device like KTP or PDL and CO_2 lasers for hypertrophic or keloidal scars with prominent vasculature. Since the channels created by the fractional device also enable molecular drug delivery [32], subsequent application of topical filler (PLLA or hyaluronic acid) or triamcinolone injectable suspension can enhance results for atrophic and hypertrophic scars, respectively.

In conclusion, fractional CO_2 lasers provide a safe treatment modality for rehabilitation of various scar types and can be combined with other therapies for optimal scar revision.

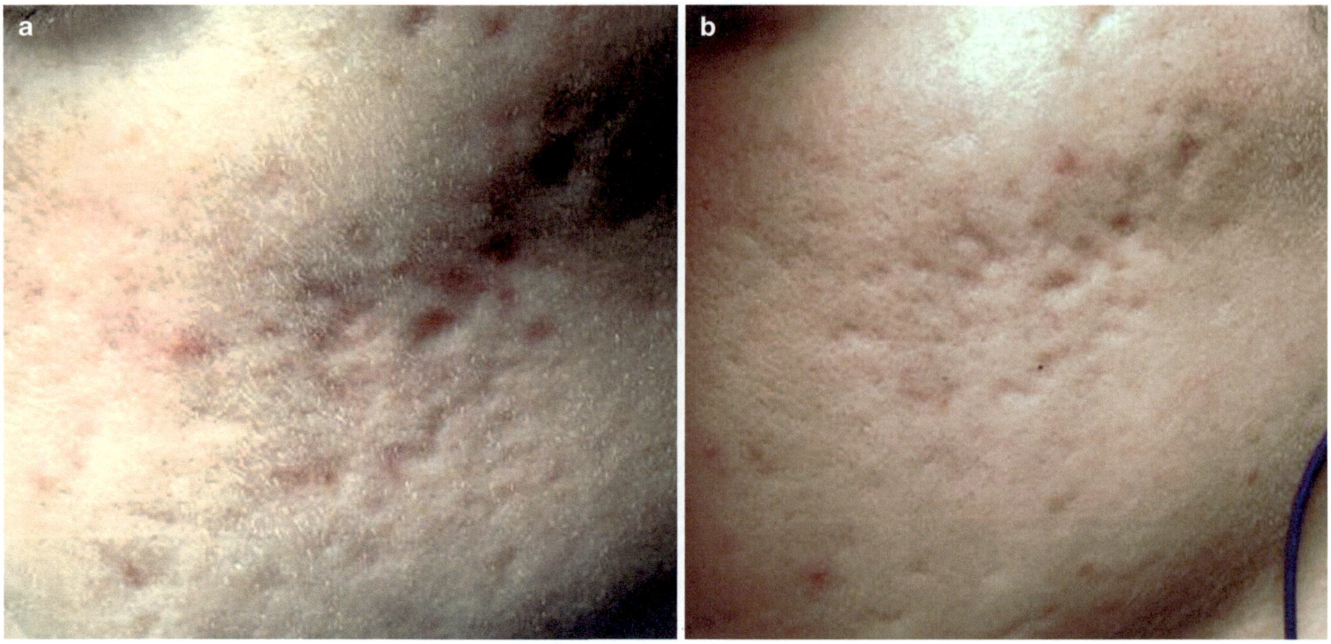

Fig. 5 (**a**) Before any treatment, erythematous, boxcar atrophic scars were noted on bilateral cheeks. (**b**) After one KTP and two CO_2 laser treatments and PLLA application, skin texture, the degree of atrophy, and erythema all improved

References

1. Heppt MV, Breuninger H, et al. Current strategies in the treatment of scars and keloids. Facial Plast Surg. 2015;31:386–95.
2. Van Drooge AM, Vrijman C, et al. A randomized controlled pilot study on ablative fractional CO_2 laser for consecutive patients presenting with various scar types. Dermatol Surg. 2015;41(3):371–7.
3. Tanzi EL, Alster TS. Laser treatment of scars. Skin Therapy Lett. 2004;9:4–7.
4. El-Zawahry BM, Sobhi RM, et al. Ablative CO_2 fractional resurfacing in treatment of thermal burn scars: an open-label controlled clinical and histopathological study. J Cosmet Dermatol. 2015;14:324–31.
5. Vrijman C, van Drooge AM, et al. Laser and intense pulsed light therapy for the treatment of hypertrophic scars: a systematic review. Br J Dermatol. 2011;165:934–42.
6. Reish RG, Eriksson E. Scars: a review of emerging and currently available therapies. Plast Reconstr Surg. 2008;122:1068–78.
7. Rkein A, Ozog D, Waibel JS. Treatment of atrophic scars with fractionated laser facilitating delivery of topically applied poly-L-lactic acid. Dermatol Surg. 2014;40:624–31.
8. Khatri KA, Mahoney DL, McCartney MJ. Laser scar revision: a review. J Cosmet Laser Ther. 2011;13:54–63.
9. Chapas AM, Brightman L, et al. Successful treatment of acneiform scarring with CO_2 ablative fractional resurfacing. Lasers Surg Med. 2008;40:381–6.
10. Ozog DM, Liu A, Chaffins M, et al. Evaluation of clinical results, histological architecture, and collagen expression following treatment of mature burn scars with a fractional carbon dioxide laser. JAMA Dermatol. 2013;149(1):50–7.
11. Laubach HJ, Tannous Z, et al. Skin responses to fractional photothermolysis. Lasers Surg Med. 2006;38:142–9.
12. Orringer JS, Voorhees JJ, et al. Dermal matrix remodeling after nonablative laser therapy. J Am Acad Dermatol. 2005;53:775–82.
13. Giordano CN, Ozog D. Microstructural and molecular considerations in the treatment of scars with ablative fractional lasers. Semin Cutan Med Surg. 2015;34:7–12.
14. Connolly KL, Chaffins M, Ozog D. Vascular patterns in mature hypertrophic burn scars treated with fractional CO_2 laser. Lasers Surg Med. 2014;46(8):597–600.
15. Verhaeghe E, Ongenaf K, et al. Nonablative fractional laser resurfacing for the treatment of hypertrophic scars: a randomized controlled trial. Dermatol Surg. 2013;39:426–34.
16. Henderson DL, Cromwell TA, Mes LG. Argon and carbon dioxide laser treatment of hypertrophic and keloid scars. Lasers Surg Med. 1984;3(4):271–7.
17. Apfelberg DB, Maser MR, Lash H, et al. Preliminary results of argon and carbon dioxide laser treatment of keloid scars. Lasers Surg Med. 1984;4(3):283–90.
18. Alster TS, Lewis AB, Rosenbach A. Laser scar revision: comparison of CO_2 laser vaporization with and without simultaneous pulse dye laser treatment. Dermatol Surg. 1998;24(12):1299–302.
19. Haedersal M. Fractional ablative CO_2 laser resurfacing improves a thermal burn scar. J Eur Acad Dermatol Venereol. 2009;23:1340–1.
20. Waibel J, Beer K. Ablative fractional laser resurfacing for the treatment of a third-degree burn. J Drugs Dermatol. 2009;8(3):294–7.
21. Qu L, Liu A, Li Z, et al. Clinical and molecular effects on mature burn scars after treatment with a fractional CO_2 laser. Lasers Surg Med. 2012;44:517–24.
22. Anderson RR, Donelan MB, Hivnor C, et al. Laser treatment of traumatic scars with an emphasis of ablative fractional laser resurfacing: a consensus report. JAMA Dermatol. 2014;150(2):187–93.
23. Azzam OA, Bassiouny DA, et al. Treatment of hypertrophic scars and keloids by fractional carbon dioxide laser: a clinical, histological, and immunohistochemical study. Lasers Med Sci. 2015; https://doi.org/10.1007/s10103-015-1824-4.
24. Nicoletti G, de Francesco F, Mele CM, et al. Clinical and histologic effects from CO2 laser treatment of keloids. Lasers Surg Med. 2013;28:957–64.
25. Nanni CA, Alster TS. Complications of carbon dioxide laser resurfacing. An evaluation of 500 patients. Dermatol Surg. 1998;24(3):315–20.
26. Bernstein LJ, Kauvar AN, et al. The short- and long-term side effects of carbon dioxide laser resurfacing. Dermatol Surg. 1997;23(7):519–25.

27. Nilforoushzadeh MA, Minaravesh S, et al. Comparison the efficacy of ablative CO_2 laser and fractional CO_2 laser on the healing of cutaneous leishmaniasis scars. Adv Biomed Res. 2014;3:259. https://doi.org/10.4103/2277-9175.148231.
28. Weiss ET, Chapas A, et al. Successful treatment of atrophic postoperative and traumatic scarring with carbon dioxide ablative fractional resurfacing: quantitative volumetric scar improvement. Arch Dermatol. 2010;146(2):133–40.
29. Lee JB, Chung WG, et al. Focal treatment of acne scars with trichloroacetic acid: chemical reconstruction of skin scars method. Dermatol Surg. 2002;28(11):1017–21.
30. Majid I, Imran S. Fractional CO_2 laser resurfacing as monotherapy in the treatment of atrophic acne scars. J Cutan Aesthet Surg. 2014;7(2):87–92.
31. Waibel JS, Wulkan AJ, Shumaker PR. Treatment of hypertrophic scars using laser and laser assisted corticosteroid delivery. Lasers Surg Med. 2013;45:135–40.
32. Sklar LR, Burnett CT, Waibel JS, et al. Laser assisted drug delivery: a review of an evolving technology. Lasers Surg Med. 2014;46:249–62.
33. van Drooge AM, Vrijman C, van der Veen W, Wolkerstorfer A. A randomized controlled pilot study on ablative fractional CO_2 laser for consecutive patients presenting with various types. Dermatol Surg. 2015;41(3):371–7.
34. Shumaker PR, Kwan JM, et al. Functional improvements in traumatic scars and scar contractures using an ablative fractional laser protocol. J Trauma Acute Care Surg. 2012;73(2):116–21.
35. Krakowski AC, Goldenberg A, et al. Ablative fractional laser resurfacing helps treat restrictive pediatric scar contractures. Pediatrics. 2014;134(6):e1700–5.
36. Kroonen L, Shumaker PR, et al. Treatment of split-thickness skin graft-related forearm scar contractures with a carbon dioxide laser protocol: 3 case reports. J Hand Surg. 2013;38(11):2165–8.
37. Nicholson CL, Hamzavi I, Ozog DM. Rapid healing of chronic ulcerations and improvement in range of motion after fractional carbon dioxide (CO_2) treatment after CO_2 excision of the hidradenitis suppurativa axillary lesions: a case report. JAAD Case Rep. 2016;2:4–6.
38. Shumaker PR, Kwan JM, et al. Rapid healing of scar-associated chronic wounds after ablative fractional resurfacing. Arch Dermatol. 2012;48(11):1289–93.
39. Krakowski AC, Diaz L, et al. Healing of chronic wounds with adjunctive ablative fractional laser resurfacing in two pediatric patients. Lasers Surg Med. 2016;48(2):166–9. https://doi.org/10.1002/lsm.22398.
40. Ozog DM, Moy RL. Discussing fractional carbon dioxide laser and other physical treatments for scar prevention with patients. JAMA Dermatol. 2015;151(8):815–6.
41. Ozog DM, Moy RL. A randomized split-scar study of intraoperative treatment of surgical wound edges to minimize scarring. Arch Dermatol. 2011;147(9):1108–10.
42. Jung JY, Jeong JJ, et al. Early postoperative treatment of thyroidectomy scars using a fractional carbon dioxide laser. Dermatol Surg. 2011;37:217–23.
43. Lee SH, Zheng Z, Roh RM. Early postoperative treatment of surgical scars using a fractional carbon dioxide laser: a split-scar, evaluator-blinded study. Dermatol Surg. 2013;39(8):1190–6.
44. Sobanko JF, Vachiramon V, et al. Early postoperative single treatment ablative fractional lasing of mohs micrographic surgery facial scars: a split-scar, evaluator-blinded study. Lasers Surg Med. 2015;47:1–5.
45. Waibel JS, Hivnor C. Chapter 11- Resurfacing. In: Kevyan N, editor. Handbook of lasers in dermatology. 1st ed. New York: Springer; 2014. p. 166–9.
46. Lowe NE, Lask G, Griffin ME. Laser skin resurfacing. Pre and post treatment guidelines. Dermatol Surg. 1995;21:1017–9.
47. Sobanko JF, Miller CJ, Alster TS. Topical anesthetics for dermatologic procedures: a review. Dermatol Surg. 2012;38:709–21.
48. Metelitsa AI, Alster TS. Fractionated laser skin resurfacing treatment complications: a review. Dermatol Surg. 2010;36:299–306.
49. Avram MM, Tope ED, Yu T, et al. Hypertrophic scarring of the neck following ablative fractional carbon dioxide resurfacing. Lasers Surg Med. 2009;41:185–8.
50. Ramsdell WM. Fractional carbon dioxide laser resurfacing. Semin Plast Surg. 2012;26:125–30.
51. Ultrapulse brochure. Lumenis. Available at: http://partnerzone.lumenis.com/DesktopModules/Bring2mind/DMX/Download.aspx?Command=Core_Download&EntryId=11314&PortalId=0&TabId=386. Accessed 12 Dec 2015.
52. Goldman MP, Roberts TL III, Skover G, et al. Optimizing wound healing in the face after laser abrasion. J Am Acad Dermatol. 2002;46(3):399–407.
53. Batra RS, Ort RJ, Jacob C, et al. Evaluation of a silicone occlusive dressing after laser skin resurfacing. Arch Dermatol. 2001;137(10):1317–21.
54. Alster TS, West TB. Effect of topical vitamin C on postoperative carbon dioxide laser resurfacing erythema. Dermatol Surg. 1998;24(3):331–4.
55. Waibel JS, Mi QS, Ozog D, et al. Laser-assisted delivery of vitamin C, vitamin E, and ferulic acid formula serum decreases fractional laser postoperative recovery by increased beta-fibroblast growth factor expression. Lasers Surg Med. 2015; https://doi.org/10.1002/lsm.22448. [Epub ahead of print].
56. Weiss RA, McDaniel DH, et al. Clinical experience with light-emitting diode (LED) photomodulation. Dermatol Surg. 2005;31(9):1199–205.
57. Alster TS, Wanitphakdeedecha R. Improvement of postfractional laser erythema with light-emitting diode photomodulation. Dermatol Surg. 2009;35(5):813–5.
58. Manstien D, Herron GS, Sink RK, et al. Fractional photothermolysis: a new concept for cutaneous remodeling using microscopic patterns of thermal injury. Lasers Surg Med. 2004;34:426–38.

Pulsed Dye Laser Treatment for the Treatment of Hypertrophic Burns Scarring

Mark Brewin and Kayvan Shokrollahi

1 Introduction

Hypertrophic scarring is often seen to occur where the injury affects the reticular dermis and, in particular, after a deep dermal or full-thickness burn [1]. Their formation results from alterations in the sequential process of wound healing, which normally proceeds in three stages:

- Inflammation
- Proliferation
- Remodelling

They are characterised by proliferation of dermal tissue with excessive deposition of fibroblast-derived extracellular matrix proteins and by persistent fibrosis and inflammation. Hypertrophic scars are generally defined as elevated, firm and erythematous. They can also be both pruritic or itchy, and painful or tender. The scars are characterised by a diffuse redness that results from a proliferation of capillary vessels inherent to chronic inflammation [2].

These scars have a rapid growth phase for up to 6 months, and then gradually regresses over a period of a few years, sometimes leading to flat scars with no further symptoms [3, 4]. It has been found that an increase in scar hypertrophy usually occurs between 6 and 12 months after the burn injury and has a tendency to regress during the maturation phase between 18 and 24 months after injury [5]. Scars mature during a period of at least 1 year and can show flattening, softening and re-pigmentation without any physical manipulation [6]. However, some scars persist and cause extended problematic management of many aspects such as functionality, erythema, pruritus and aesthesis.

M. Brewin (✉)
Salisbury Laser Clinic, Salisbury NHS Foundation Trust, Salisbury, Wiltshire, UK
e-mail: mark.brewin@salisbury.nhs.uk

K. Shokrollahi
Burns and Plastic Surgery Unit, Whiston Hospital, Liverpool, UK

2 Review of the Evidence

2.1 Pulsed Dye Laser for Hypertrophic Scars

PDL technologies have been tested to either prevent or treat hypertrophic scars by selective destruction of scar microvasculature through the process of targeted photothermolysis [7]. Other theories of the mechanism by which PDL may achieve clinical effectiveness in their treatment include by the decreased cellular activity resultant from laser-induced anoxia or through collagenolysis by laser stimulation of cytokine release [8]. Healing may also be induced by the effects of histamine on dermal collagen [9].

Historically, the 585-nm PDL has been shown to effectively improve the pliability and texture of hypertrophic scars, as well as reduce the erythema and the associated symptoms of pain and pruritus [10], though some studies do not concur [11, 12]. Several studies from the former research group have demonstrated significant clinical improvement to a variety of scars [13–15].

2.2 Early Intervention

The primary mechanism of PDL therapy is to target the destruction of small blood vessels by photothermolysis. Previous studies have indeed shown that laser treatment of scars has had good results in reduction of erythema but with varying degrees of success for other aspects of scarring. It has been hypothesised that treatment during the early stages of wound healing or the inflammatory stage, before scar for-

K. Shokrollahi (ed.), *Laser Management of Scars*, https://doi.org/10.1007/978-3-030-52919-2_6

mation, could avoid these further aspects [16, 17]. Indeed, treatment options should be considered early in patients that are identified as prone to scarring.

It is suggested that pulsed dye laser should be used in the treatment of hypertrophic scars resulting from burns wounds. If these scars are exposed to PDL laser light at an early stage of maturation, i.e. less than 6 months since wound healing, then the process of scar healing could be both improved and accelerated [16, 17, 8, 18, 19]. In this way, the severity of the outcome of hypertrophic scars could be reduced.

Effective strategies for both the prevention and treatment of hypertrophic scars remain elusive. The transition of intervention protocol from that of prevention to that of treatment can only occur once the diagnosis of a scar is made, although either can be considered similar both practically and in their concept. Early intervention was deemed by an international panel of experts to be much more efficient in preventing hypertrophic scars rather than in treating them [18]. As our knowledge of wound evolution increases, prevention and treatment should become differentiated. The most successful treatment of a hypertrophic scar may be achieved when the scar is immature, though there is not yet sufficient evidence to support this rationale.

2.3 Previous Studies

Dierickx et al. [8] reviewed the effect of using 585-nm PDL on erythematous and hypertrophic scars occurring after surgical procedures. They reported that an incidence of total resolution of 12% and an improvement of 62% was seen after an average of 2.2 treatments in non-facial areas for scars over 1 year of age. However, a 25% incidence of total resolution over an average of 2.5 treatments with an average improvement of 81% for scars on non-facial areas of less than 1 year old was observed. The paper suggests that a minimum of four treatments at an interval of 4–8 weeks would be required for a clear improvement in objective clinical measurement and it advocates treatment within the first few weeks of injury to prevent scar proliferation.

A study in Hong Kong has looked at the difference between treatment and prevention using 585-nm PDL for hypertrophic scars [20]. The patients were divided into two groups according to the age of the scar at first treatment; either more or less than 6 months old. The patient cohort was 29 Asian patients with 35 scars. The majority of these scars were a result of surgery, 88%, as opposed to burns, 6%. Treatment efficacy was tested subjectively through a patient questionnaire and objectively using sonography for scar thickness, a cutometer for viscoelasticity and a spectrophotometer for colour. Significant symptomatic improvement as assessed by patient questionnaire was seen in both groups, whereas there was no significant change in thickness and pliability in each group compared to the untreated sites. However, there was significant improvement in skin lightness seen in the treatment group despite there being no reduction in redness. This study concludes that PDL therapy may not be useful for surgical scars in Asian patients.

Further to this, a 585-nm PDL treatment study for burns scars looked at the effect on old and new scars according to whether they were more or less than 3 months old [11]. No difference was found in clinical behaviour or scar assessment between groups although the authors noted that the study size was small, with 13 new and 25 old scars. However, they included the use or EMLA or Ametop for analgesia and this is known to reduce the blood flow to the treated area. This would lessen the effect of destroying blood vessels within the scar. The study method selected was intra-scar where the scar area was divided into two equal halves, treatment and control. There is some argument that the treatment would also affect the control part of the scar. The treatment was also carried out at a relatively low fluence of 5–6 Jcm^{-2} with a small spot size of 5 mm. They postulated that the treatment may be improved with the use of cooling and the matching of the pulse duration to the microvascular nature of the vessels in a burns scar. A pulse width of 100 ms was suggested to match the vessel diameter range of 3.3–14.6 μm, yet no further study has explored this pulse width. They concluded that it is likely that the beneficial effects demonstrated thus far result from changes to the chemical signals that regulate the scar growth and symptoms.

In another study, prophylactic treatment of burn wounds with PDL in the first 3 months has been shown to result in a reduction in scar formation. Six scars on five patients were treated and seen to resolve faster than non-treated control areas [21]. Two treatments of 585-nm PDL at 6-week intervals were used with the same laser (Chromos 585, SLS, Wales) at a higher energy setting of 6–9 J cm^{-2}. Again, the intra-scar method was used for the control. The scars were clinically assessed for colour, contour, texture, distortion and finish using the Manchester Scar Scale [22]. The treated areas showed better scarring at 6 weeks and 3 months yet there was no significant difference at 6 months and no apparent long-term benefit. In this way, it was shown to be effective in hastening the resolution of scarring and therefore its use should be considered early in the scar management protocol. This preliminary study did not show any difference in the long term but the study population was small.

Previously, McCraw et al. [23] also reported in a preliminary study that, for 106 patients on 171 sites treated within 3 weeks of injury, post-operative hypertrophic scars showed fast resolution in both stiffness and erythema and that there was an overall improvement in scar quality. Here, a 585-nm PDL was also used with lower energies of 2.5–4.5 J cm^{-2} with a 10 mm spot. No control was used in their study and it was not acknowledged that hypertrophic scars tend to improve with time.

A recent systematic review of laser and intense pulsed light (IPL) therapy for the treatment of hypertrophic scars showed a low level of efficacy for 585-nm PDL as opposed to a moderate level for 595-nm PDL [24]. In their paper, little significant evidence was found for the efficacy of other lasers and therefore further research using 595-nm PDL is deemed necessary. However, their review had focussed on the treatment of scars that were at least 6 months old as they had been interested in the treatment, rather than prevention, of mature hypertrophic scars. Nevertheless, it may be prudent to perform further testing of the 595-nm PDL in hypertrophic scar therapy.

3 Treatment Methodology

The PDL protocols previously used have adopted an energy of around 2.5–9 J cm^{-2} with a 5–10 mm spot. It is considered that higher fluences of 6–9 J cm^{-2} should be selected using a larger spot of 10 mm. The commonly used pulse duration has been 0.5 ms. There is a theoretical argument for the further shortening of this variable; however, the shortest pulse durations for the two commercially available PDLs: Cynergy (Cynosure, Westford, MA, USA) and Vbeam Perfecta (Syneron Candela, CA, USA) are 0.5 and 0.45 ms, respectively. In general, success has been shown when two to three treatments have been performed at intervals of around 6 weeks. The scar should be at an immature stage at below 6 months old, and the study sample would ideally have a skin type of Fitzpatrick scale I–IV in order to avoid adverse effects.

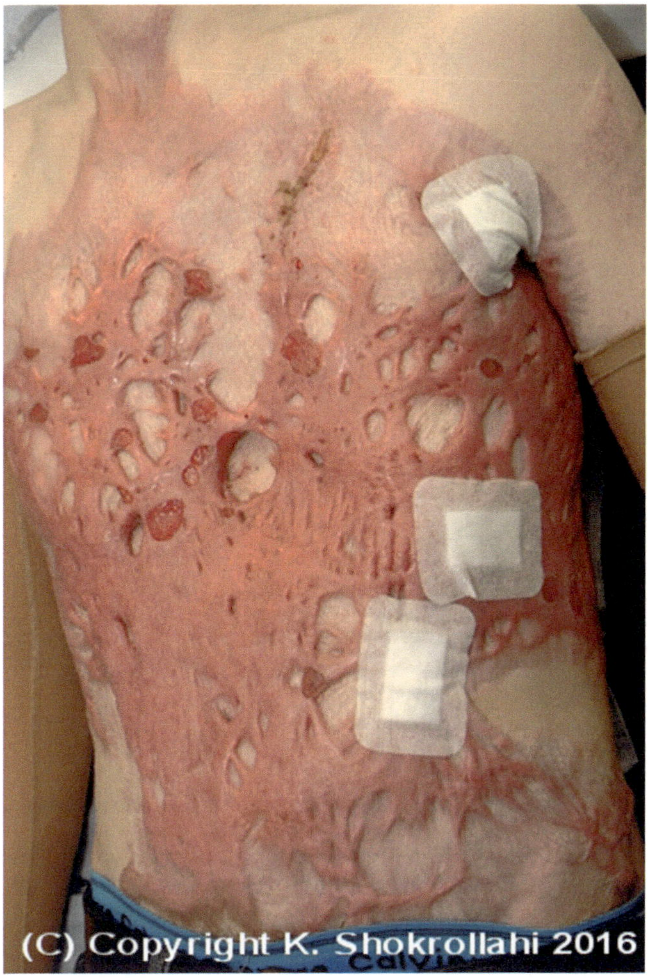

Fig. 1 Hypertrophic chest scars from complicated full-thickness burns, pre-laser treatment (patient of KS). Copyright K. Shokrollahi 2016

4 Case Example

Florid hypertrophic scarring on the chest of a burn survivor is demonstrated in Fig. 1. The nature of the hypertrophic scarring is severe due to the delayed nature of the healing as a consequence of pseudomonas infection and prolonged illness from pneumonia on intensive care prior to recovery.

Seven sessions of mainly pulsed dye laser have had a considerable impact on the hypertrophy and erythema of the scars over 9 months (Fig. 2). Some carbon dioxide laser has also been used for specific areas of thickened scarring.

4.1 Lasers Settings

Laser: Cynosure Cynergy Laser (Combined PDL and ND:YAG laser).

Laser used: PDL.
Spot size: 12 mm.
Fluence: 0.5 ms.
Cooling: yes (cryo air blower).
Contact gel: yes (ultrasound gel).

5 Discussion

The pulsed dye laser has one of the longest track records in the treatment of hypertrophic scarring and a good evidence base. Hypertrophic scars have a tendency to improve with time which adds a tier of difficulty when demonstrating the positive effects of PDL. Nevertheless, the evidence for accelerated improvements of hypertrophic scarring has been sufficient for it to have been widely adopted as a modality at the heart of hypertrophic scar management.

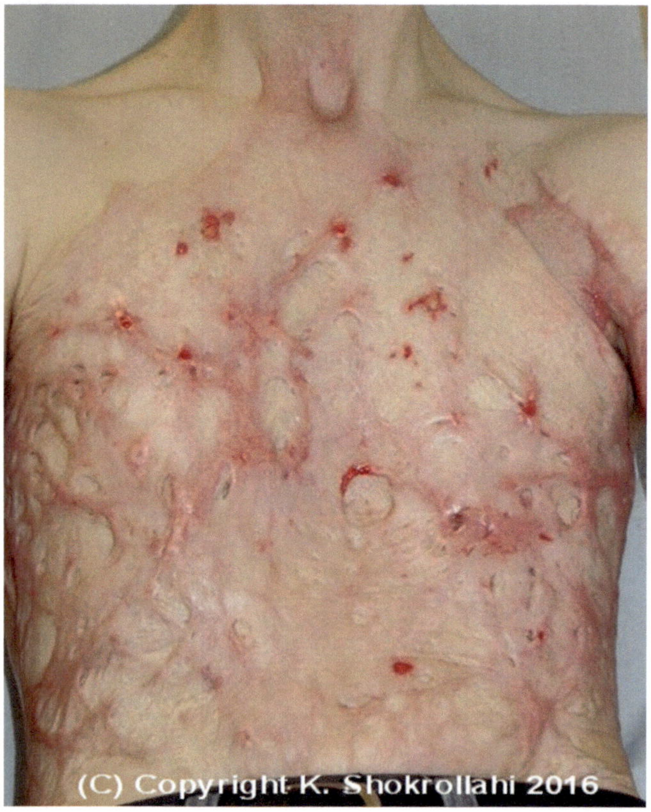

Fig. 2 Hypertrophic burns scars of the chest 9 months after seven sessions of pulsed dye laser (patient treated by KS). Copyright K. Shokrollahi 2016

References

1. Singh V, Devgan L, Bhat S, Milner SM. The pathogenesis of burn wound conversion. Ann Plast Surg. 2007;59(1):109–15.
2. Clark J, Leung K, Cheng J, Leung PC. The hypertrophic scar and microcirculation properties. Burns. 1996;22(6):447–50.
3. Alster T, Handrick C. Laser treatment of hypertrophic scars, keloids, and striae. Semin Cutan Med Surg. 2000;19(4):287–92.
4. Gauglitz GG, Korting HC, Pavicic T, Ruzicka T, Jeschke MG. Hypertrophic scarring and keloids: pathomechanisms and current and emerging treatment strategies. Mol Med. 2011;17(1–2):113.
5. Oliveira GV, Chinkes D, Mitchell C, Oliveras G, Hawkins HK, Herndon DN. Objective assessment of burn scar vascularity, erythema, pliability, thickness, and planimetry. Dermatol Surg. 2005;31(1):48–58.
6. Reish RG, Eriksson E. Scars: a review of emerging and currently available therapies. Plast Reconstr Surg. 2008;122(4):1068–78.
7. Reiken S, Wolfort S, Berthiaume F, Compton C, Tompkins R, Yarmush M. Control of hypertrophic scar growth using selective photothermolysis. Lasers Surg Med. 1997;21(1):7–12.
8. Dierickx CC, Goldman MP, Fitzpatrick RE. Laser treatment of erythematous/hypertrophic and pigmented scars in 26 patients. Plast Reconstr Surg. 1995;95(1):84–90.
9. Alster TS, Williams CM. Treatment of keloid sternotomy scars with 585 nm flashlamp-pumped pulsed-dye laser. Lancet. 1995;345(8959):1198–200.
10. Alster T, Nanni C. Pulsed dye laser treatment of hypertrophic burn scars. Plast Reconstr Surg. 1998;102(6):2190–5.
11. Allison K, Kiernan M, Waters R, Clement R. Pulsed dye laser treatment of burn scars. Burns. 2003;29(3):207–13.
12. Wittenburg G, Fabian B, Bogomilsky J, Schultz L, Rudner E, Chaffins M, et al. Prospective, single-blind, randomized, controlled study to assess the efficacy of the 585-nm flashlamp-pumped pulsed-dye laser and silicone gel sheeting in hypertrophic scar treatment. Arch Dermatol. 1999;135(9):1049–55.
13. Alster T. Improvement of erythematous and hypertrophic scars by the 585-nm flashlamp-pumped pulsed dye laser. Ann Plast Surg. 1994;32(2):186–90.
14. Alster TS, McMeekin T. Improvement of facial acne scars by the 585 nm flashlamp-pumped pulsed dye laser. J Am Acad Dermatol. 1996;35(1):79–81.
15. Alster T, Zaulyanov-Scanlon L. Laser scar revision: a review. Dermatol Surg. 2007;33(2):131–40.
16. Bloemen MCT, van der Veer WM, Ulrich MMW, van Zuijlen PPM, Niessen FB, Middelkoop E. Prevention and curative management of hypertrophic scar formation. Burns. 2009;35(4):463–75.
17. Leclère FM, Mordon SR. Twenty-five years of active laser prevention of scars: what have we learned? J Cosmet Laser Ther. 2010;12(5):227–34.
18. Mustoe TA, Cooter RD, Gold MH, Hobbs FR, Ramelet A, Shakespeare P, et al. International clinical recommendations on scar management. Plast Reconstr Surg. 2002;110(2):560–71.
19. Gold MH, McGuire M, Mustoe TA, Pusic A, Sachdev M, Waibel J, et al. Updated international clinical recommendations on scar management: part 2—algorithms for scar prevention and treatment. Dermatol Surg. 2014;40(8):825–31.
20. Chan HH, Wong DS, Ho WS, Lam LK, Wei W. The use of pulsed dye laser for the prevention and treatment of hypertrophic scars in Chinese persons. Dermatol Surg. 2004;30(7):987–94.
21. Liew SH, Murison M, Dickson WA. Prophylactic treatment of deep dermal burn scar to prevent hypertrophic scarring using the pulsed dye laser: a preliminary study. Ann Plast Surg. 2002;49(5):472–5.
22. Beausang E, Floyd H, Dunn KW, Orton C, Ferguson MWJ. A new quantitative scale for clinical scar assessment. Plast Reconstr Surg. 1998;102(6):1954–61.
23. McCraw J, McCraw J, McMellin A, Bettencourt N. Prevention of unfavorable scars using early pulse dye laser treatments: a preliminary report. Ann Plast Surg. 1999;42(1):7–14.
24. Vrijman C, van Drooge AM, Limpens J, Bos JD, van der Veen JPW, Spuls PI, et al. Laser and intense pulsed light therapy for the treatment of hypertrophic scars: a systematic review: laser and IPL therapy for hypertrophic scars. Br J Dermatol. 2011;165(5):934–42.

Further Reading

Bailey JK. Multimodal quantitative analysis of early pulsed-dye laser treatment of scars at a pediatric burn hospital. Dermatol Surg. (2012);38(9):1490–6.

Brewin MP, Lister TS. Prevention or treatment of hypertrophic burn scarring: a review of when and how to treat with the pulsed dye laser. Burns. 2014;40:797–804.

Gladsjo J, Jiang S. Treatment of surgical scars using a 595-nm pulsed dye laser using purpuric and nonpurpuric parameters: a comparative study. Dermatol Surg. 2014;40(2):118–26.

Hultman CS, Edkins RE, Wu C, Calvert CT, Cairns BA. Prospective, before-after cohort study to assess the efficacy of laser therapy on hypertrophic burn scars. Ann Plast Surg. 2013;70:521–26.

Karmisholt KE. et al. Early laser intervention to reduce scar formation - a systematic review. J Eur Acad Dermatol Venereol. JEADV 2018;32:1099–10.

Monstrey S. et al. Updated scar management practical guidelines: non-invasive and invasive measures. J Plast Reconstr Aesthet Surg. 2014;67:1017–25.

Richardson C, Upton D, Rippon M. Treatment for wound pruritus following burns. J Wound Care. 2014;23(5):227–3.

Long-Pulsed 1064-nm Nd:YAG Laser Treatment for Keloids and Hypertrophic Scars

Rei Ogawa

1 Introduction

Keloids and hypertrophic scars are fibroproliferative disorders of the skin that are caused by abnormal healing of injured or irritated skin [1]. Both disorders have similar histological features: the epidermis and the papillary layer of the dermis are almost normal apart from slight inflammation and the only abnormality is in the reticular layer of the dermis [2]. While keloids typically exhibit marked hyalinized collagen deposition as a result of prolonged and strong inflammation, this feature is less pronounced in hypertrophic scars [3]. Thus, it is possible that hypertrophic scars and keloids are manifestations of the same fibroproliferative skin disorder and just differ in the intensity and duration of inflammation. These features may in turn be influenced by genetic, systemic, and local risk factors. It is possible that keloids arise largely as a result of genetic and systemic factors that promote massive and extended inflammation, while hypertrophic scars are more likely to be due to local factors. Genetic factors may include single nucleotide polymorphisms [4, 5] while systemic factors may include hypertension [6, 7], pregnancy [8, 9], hormones, and cytokines. The most important local factor is skin tension on the edges of the scar [10–12].

Our understanding of the pathogenesis of keloids and hypertrophic scars has improved markedly in the last 10 years, and these previously intractable scars are now regarded as being treatable. This has dramatically improved the quality of life of patients with these heavy scars [3]. There are many therapeutic options for keloids and hypertrophic scars, including surgery, radiation, corticosteroids, 5-fluorouracil, cryotherapy, laser therapy, anti-allergy agents, anti-inflammatory agents, bleaching creams, and make-up therapies. In terms of laser therapy, we have used long-pulsed 1064-nm Nd:YAG laser to treat keloids and hypertrophic scars and have reported its indications and limitations previously [13, 14].

R. Ogawa (✉)
Department of Plastic, Reconstructive and Aesthetic Surgery, Nippon Medical School, Tokyo, Japan
e-mail: r.ogawa@nms.ac.jp

2 Laser Therapies for Keloids and Hypertrophic Scars

Pulsed dye laser (PDL) has long been the therapy of choice for cutaneous vascular diseases, including telangiectasia, hemangioma, and vascular malformations [15–17]. It has also been used to treat keloids and hypertrophic scars because they have more blood vessels than normal skin. However, although PDL is effective for vascular diseases that affect the superficial skin layers (i.e., the epidermis and the papillary layer of the dermis), it does not penetrate deep enough to reach the deep dermal regions (i.e., the reticular layer of the dermis). Thus, PDL is not particularly effective for keloids and hypertrophic scars. By contrast, 1064-nm Nd:YAG laser reaches more deeply than PDL. As a result, it is increasingly being used to treat keloids and hypertrophic scars [13, 18–21]. It has been suggested that it acts by suppressing neovascularization and the dilatation of blood vessels.

Long-pulsed (not Q-switched) 1064-nm Nd:YAG laser plays an important role in our treatment algorithms for keloids and hypertrophic scars. This laser was developed for the treatment of vascular diseases, including inflammatory scars that exhibit neovascularization. It is also used to remove hair and to rejuvenate the skin [13]. The depth that is reached is determined by the spot size, the laser power, and the fluence: the larger the spot size, power, or fluence, the deeper the laser beam penetrates. Therefore, a large spot size and/or power are used for deep targets such as hair follicles and the blood vessels in the reticular layer of the dermis. However, since larger power increases the risk of cutaneous burn injury, the power should be determined on a case-by-case basis.

K. Shokrollahi (ed.), *Laser Management of Scars*, https://doi.org/10.1007/978-3-030-52919-2_7

3 Indications and Limitations of Long-Pulsed 1064-nm Nd:YAG Laser for Keloids and Hypertrophic Scars

Keloid and hypertrophic scar development are due to chronic inflammation of the dermis during the course of wound healing. This associates with prolonged angiogenesis and collagen production. As mentioned above, long-pulsed 1064-nm Nd:YAG laser treatment may effectively treat keloid and hypertrophic scars because it reduces their vascularity. This reduction in vascularity may in turn decrease cytokine or growth factor levels in the tissue, which then promote collagen deposition. This notion is supported by the ability of several vascularity-suppressing treatments to improve inflammation and thereby ameliorate abnormal scars. One such treatment may be compression therapy, which is widely used with heavy scars, especially for hypertrophic scars that arise from burn wounds. This therapy may force the collapse of blood vessels in the scar, thereby decreasing cytokine or growth factor levels in the tissue. Moreover, it has been suggested that radiation therapy is effective for keloids because it suppresses angiogenesis. However, studies elucidating the mechanisms underlying long-pulsed 1064-nm Nd:YAG laser treatment efficacy in abnormal scars are warranted.

Our previous study [13] suggests that repeated tension on the edges of scars that is imposed by body movements prolongs scar inflammation: we observed that the patterns of mechanical force distribution around keloids and hypertrophic scars are largely consistent with the shape of the scar. In particular, our study suggests that keloids grow into the direction of the dominant prevailing skin tension. This mechanism explains why keloids on different regions of the body adopt specific shapes, such as the butterfly on the shoulder, the dumbbell on the upper arm, and the crab's claw on the anterior chest. These observations suggest that, if scars will continue to be subjected to strong tension due to the daily movements of the body, long-pulsed 1064-nm Nd:YAG laser will not be successful. Indeed, our experience suggests that scars on less stretched areas (i.e., the face and anterior lower leg) respond better to this therapy than scars on highly stretched areas (i.e., the anterior chest wall and scapula). We also found that (1) less inflamed scars (i.e., the typical hypertrophic scar) (Figs. 1, 2, and 3)

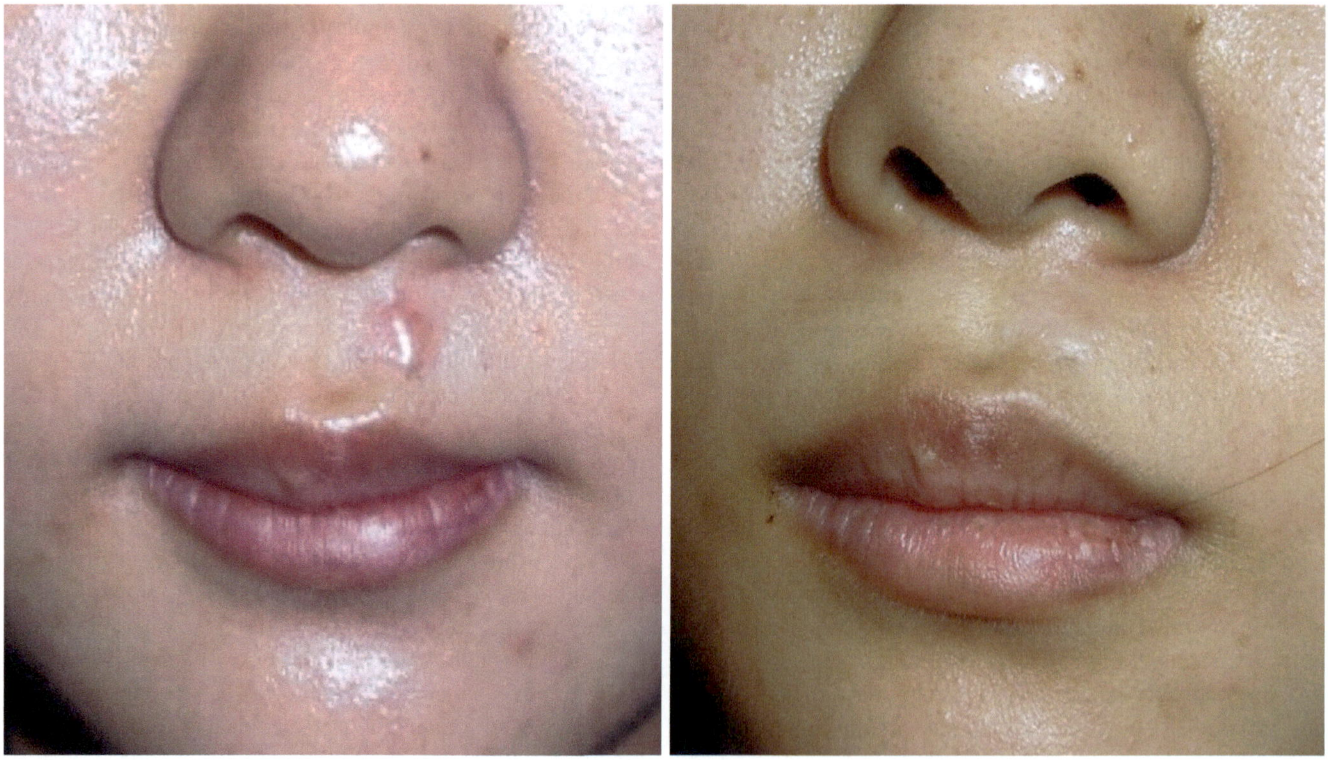

Fig. 1 Upper lip hypertrophic scar. Left: before treatment. Right: 1 year after treatment. Two years before her referral to our clinic, a 20-year-old female received an abrasion injury to her upper lip that turned into a hypertrophic scar. Long-pulsed 1064-nm Nd:YAG laser was used at the following settings: 5 mm spot diameter, 65–70 J/cm^2, 25 ms, and 2 Hz. After 1 year of this treatment, the scar continued to exhibit a textural difference but its redness and elevation had improved. (This figure is cited from reference [13] with approval from the publisher)

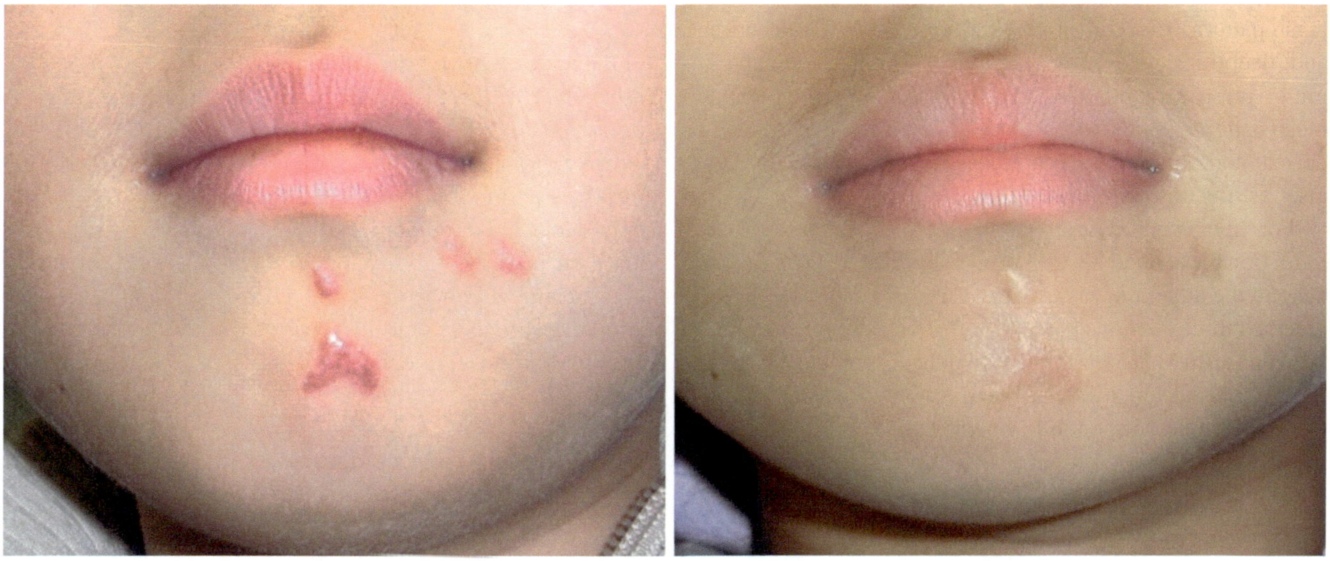

Fig. 2 Lower lip hypertrophic scar. Left: before treatment. Right: 1 year after treatment. One year before her referral to our clinic, a 11-year-old female received an abrasion injury to her lower lip that developed into hypertrophic scars. Long-pulsed 1064-nm Nd:YAG laser was used at the following settings: 5 mm spot diameter, 60–70 J/cm^2, 25 ms, and 2 Hz. After 1 year of treatment, the scars continued to display textural differences and elevation but there was clear improvement in their redness. (This figure is cited from reference [13] with approval from the publisher)

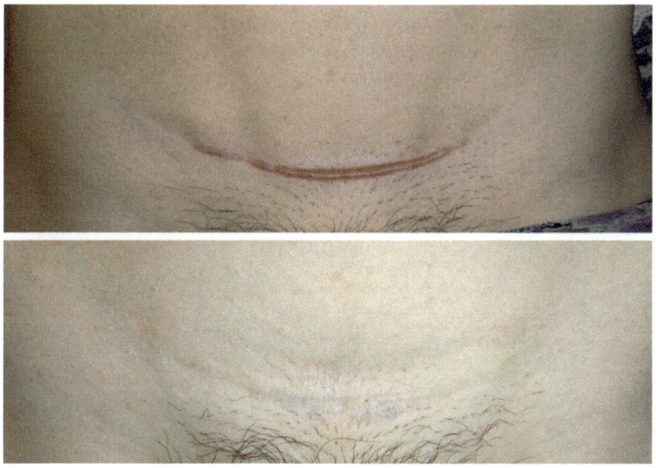

Fig. 3 Abdomen hypertrophic scar. Upper: before treatment. Lower: 1 year after treatment. Four years before her referral to our clinic, a 50-year-old female developed hypertrophic scars on her abdomen after uterine myoma surgery. Long-pulsed 1064-nm Nd:YAG laser was used at the following settings: 5 mm spot diameter, 75 J/cm^2, 25 ms, and 2 Hz. After 1 year of treatment, the scar had almost disappeared. (This figure is cited from reference [13] with approval from the publisher)

respond better than highly inflamed scars (i.e., the typical keloid) (Figs. 4, 5, and 6); (2) thinner scars respond better than thick scars; (3) small scars respond better than large scars; (4) single scars respond better than multiple scars (Fig. 7); and (5) if even a little scar redness and induration remains after long-pulsed 1064-nm Nd:YAG laser treatment, these scars are highly likely to recur.

4 Treatment Settings of Long-Pulsed 1064-nm Nd:YAG Laser for Keloids and Hypertrophic Scars

The laser should generally be applied to the skin surface with the following standard treatment settings: a spot diameter of 5 mm, an energy density of 75 J/cm^2, an exposure time per pulse of 25 ms, and a repetition rate of 2 Hz. However, in the case of the face (Figs. 1 and 2) or pediatric patients, the treatment should start with a lower energy density (60–70 J/cm^2) to reduce the possibility of a burn injury. The best way to prevent such burn injuries is to cool the tip or air cool the targeted skin before and immediately after irradiation. Each session should consist of three passes unless the patient feels strong pain at the second pass; in this case, the session should be stopped. Even if the patient feels no pain after the third pass, the session should be stopped. Local anesthesia is not necessary. However, if the patient expresses concern, anesthesia cream or tape can be used. The intervals between the sessions should generally be 2–4 weeks depending on the patient's schedule.

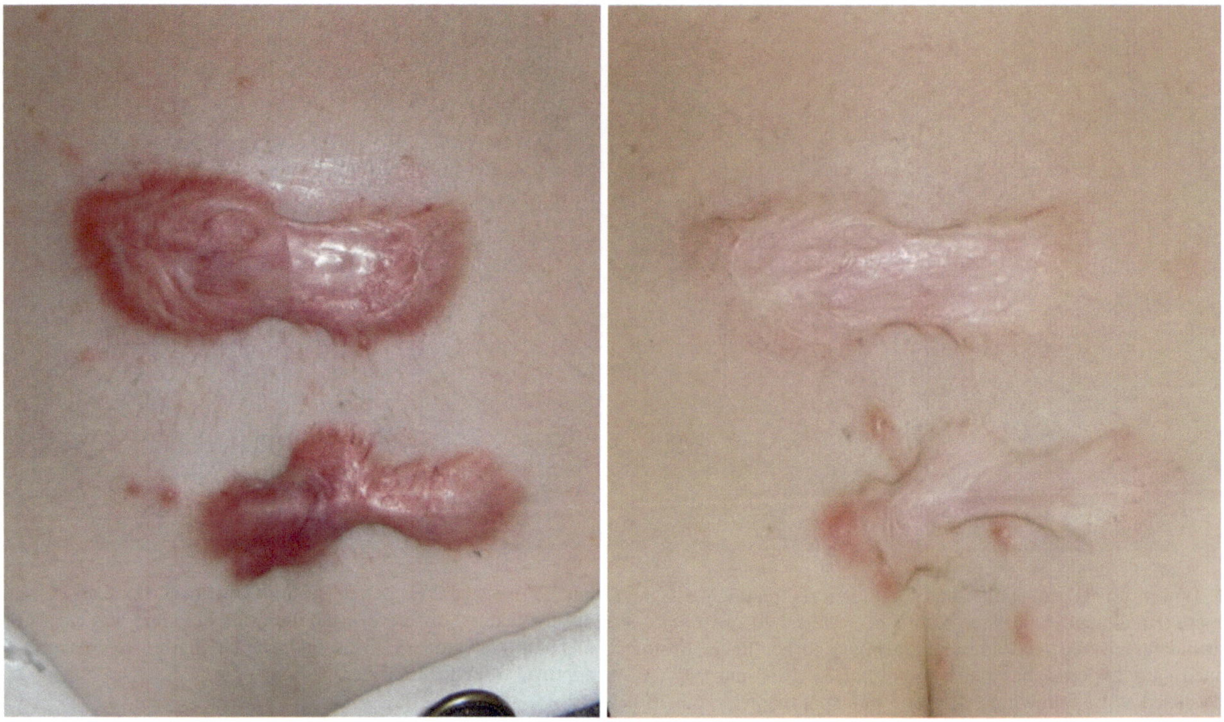

Fig. 4 Anterior chest wall keloid. Left: before treatment. Right: 1 year after treatment. Eleven years before her referral to our clinic, a 29-year-old female developed butterfly-shaped keloids on her anterior chest. Treatment with steroid ointment and tape at other clinics did not improve these scars. Long-pulsed Nd:YAG laser was used at the following settings: 5 mm spot diameter, 65–75 J/cm^2, 25 ms, and 2 Hz. After 1 year of treatment, the textural differences and elevation had improved but there was remaining redness on some parts. (This figure is cited from reference [13] with approval from the publisher)

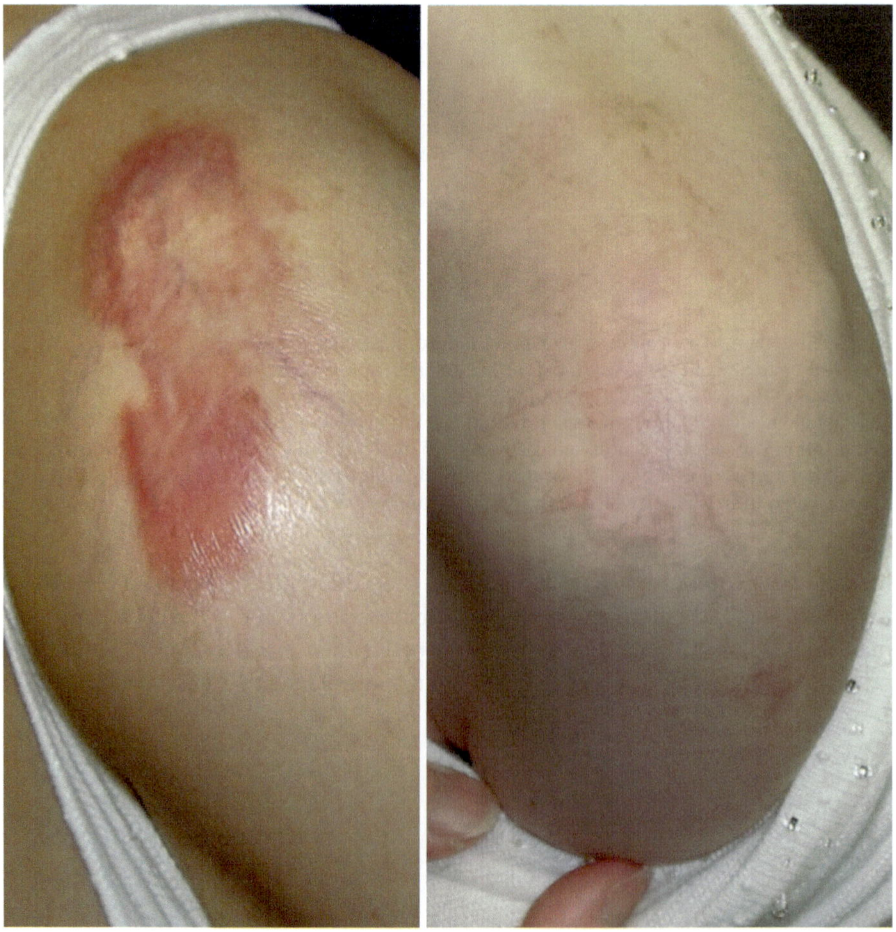

Fig. 5 Shoulder keloid. Left: before treatment. Right: 30 months after treatment. About 20 years before her referral to our clinic, a 52-year-old female developed butterfly-shaped keloids on her upper arm and shoulder. Long-pulsed 1064 nm Nd:YAG laser was used at the following settings: 5 mm spot diameter, 70–75 J/cm^2, 25 ms, and 2 Hz. After 1 year of treatment, there were clear improvements in the textural differences and elevation but there was remaining redness on some parts. There was also some capillary dilation that was the result of steroid injections in the past. (This figure is cited from reference [13] with approval from the publisher)

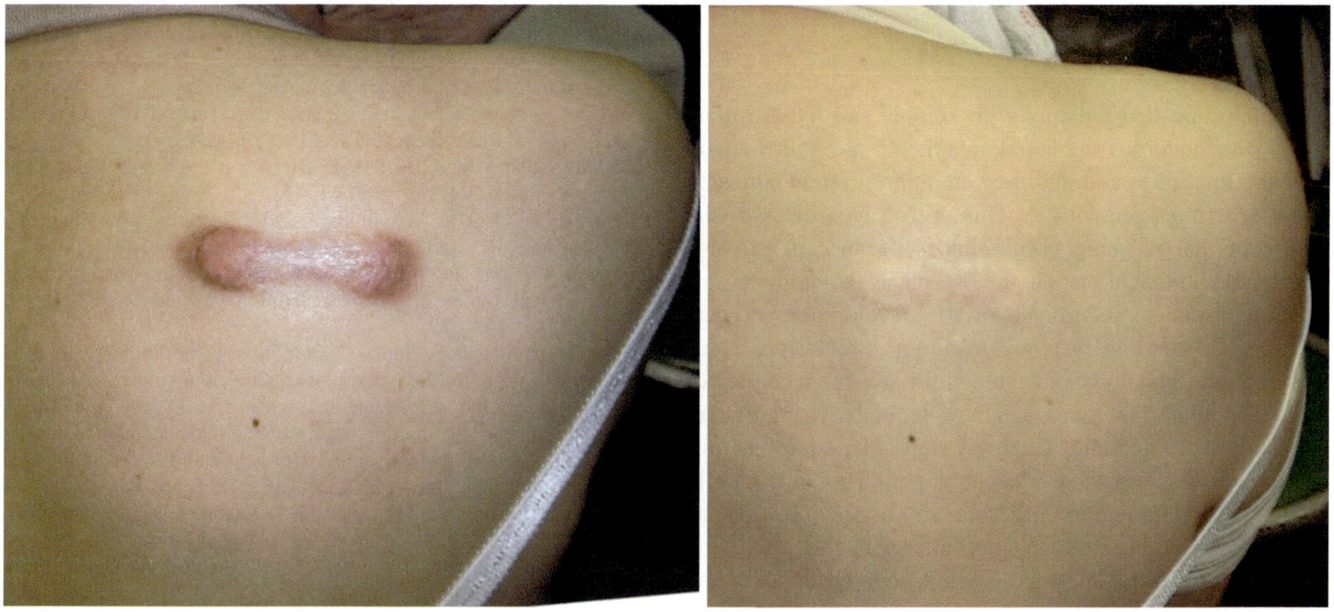

Fig. 6 Scapular keloid. Left: before treatment. Right: 3 years after treatment. About 30 years before her referral to our clinic, a 52-year-old female developed a butterfly-shaped keloid on her scapula. Steroid injections and tape at other clinics yielded little improvement. Long-pulsed 1064 nm Nd:YAG laser was used at the following settings: 5 mm spot diameter, 70–75 J/cm^2, 25 ms, and 2 Hz. After 2 years of treatment, the texture, redness, induration, and elevation of the scar had clearly improved. (This figure is cited from reference [13] with approval from the publisher)

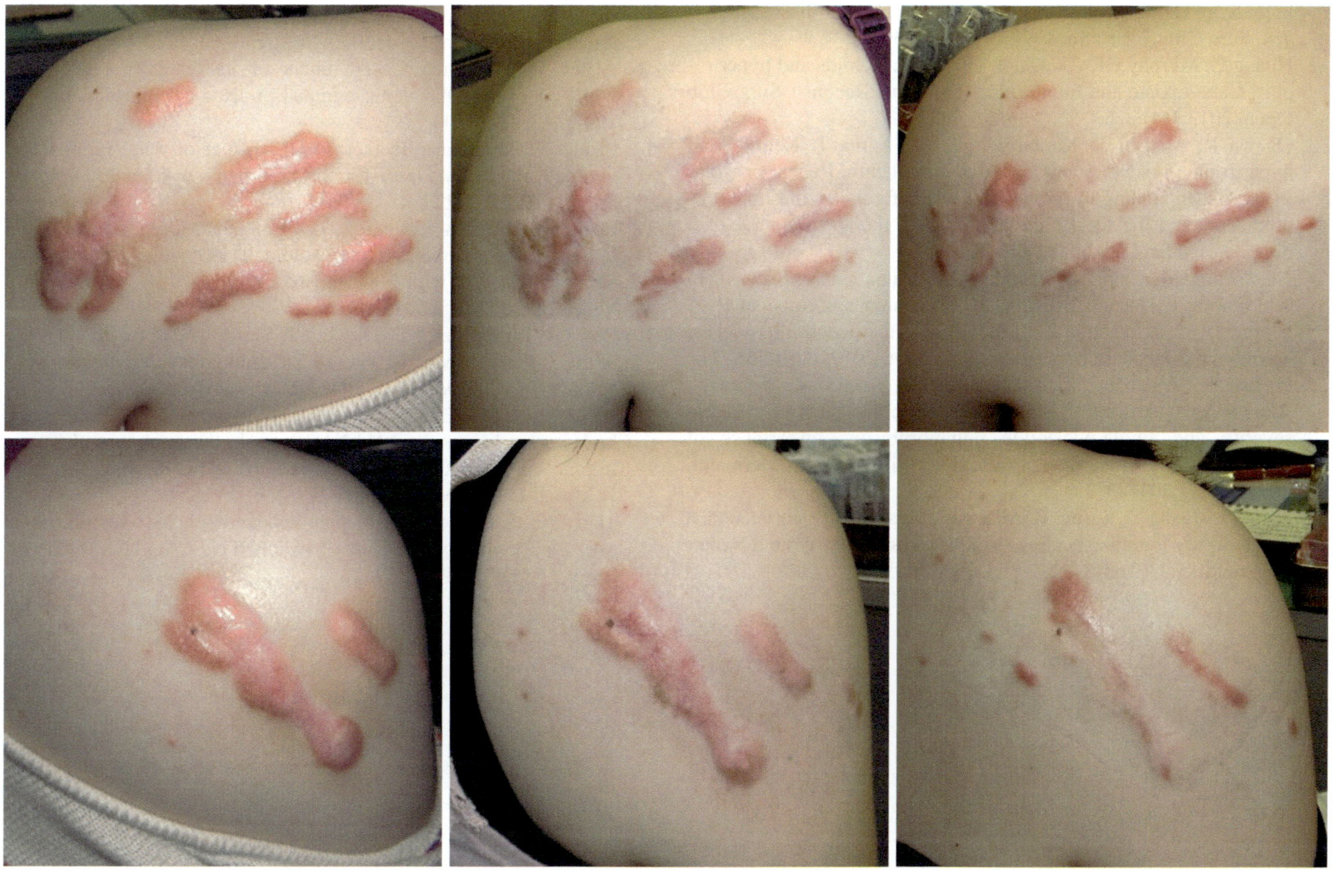

Fig. 7 Scapular keloid. Left images: before treatment. Middle images: after 1 year of treatment. Right images: after 4 years of treatment. About 30 years before her referral to our clinic, a 42-year-old female developed multiple keloids on both the left (top images) and right (bottom images) scapular areas. The keloids had been slowly increasing in size. Steroid injections and tape treatment at other clinics yielded little improvement. Long-pulsed 1064 nm Nd:YAG laser was used at the following settings: 5 mm spot diameter, 75 J/cm^2, 25 ms, and 2 Hz. Moreover, a Chinese herb (Saireito) was administered every day. After 4 years of treatment, the texture, redness, induration, and elevation of the scars have improved. However, the scars are not yet completely cured

5 Follow-Up of Keloids and Hypertrophic Scars

It is important that patients with keloids and hypertrophic scars who undergo sequential treatments are followed up over the long term and that they are appropriately educated about scar management [3]. This is true regardless of the treatment that is being used. This is because, if patients develop pathological scars in the first place, they may be particularly prone to recurrence or the development of new pathological scars in response to minor stimulation. Thus, these patients should be educated in the self-management of both their abnormal scars and new wounds. In particular, they should be encouraged to apply steroid tape/plasters during the early stages of scar development. This will rapidly reduce the inflammation in the scar and improve its appearance. Moreover, laser therapy, anti-allergy agents (including tranilast), anti-inflammatory agents, bleaching creams, and make-up therapies can be used on a case-by-case basis [3].

References

1. Tredget EE, Nedelec B, Scott PG, Ghahary A. Hypertrophic scars, keloids, and contractures. The cellular and molecular basis for therapy. Surg Clin North Am. 1997;77(3):701–30.
2. Huang C, Murphy GF, Akaishi S, Ogawa R. Keloids and hypertrophic scars: update and future directions. Plast Reconstr Surg Glob Open. 2013;1(4):e25.
3. Ogawa R, Akaishi S, Kuribayashi S, Miyashita T. Keloids and hypertrophic scars can now be cured completely: Recent progress in our understanding of the pathogenesis of keloids and hypertrophic scars and the most promising current therapeutic strategy. J Nippon Med Sch. 2016;83(2):46–53.
4. Nakashima M, Chung S, Takahashi A, Kamatani N, Kawaguchi T, Tsunoda T, Hosono N, Kubo M, Nakamura Y, Zembutsu H. A genome-wide association study identifies four susceptibility loci for keloid in the Japanese population. Nat Genet. 2010;42(9):768–71.
5. Ogawa R, Watanabe A, Than Naing B, Sasaki M, Fujita A, Akaishi S, Hyakusoku H, Shimada T. Associations between keloid severity and single-nucleotide polymorphisms: importance of rs8032158 as a biomarker of keloid severity. J Invest Dermatol. 2014;134(7):2041–3.
6. Arima J, Huang C, Rosner B, Akaishi S, Ogawa R. Hypertension: a systemic key to understanding local keloid severity. Wound Repair Regen. 2015;23(2):213–21.
7. Huang C, Ogawa R. The link between hypertension and pathological scarring: does hypertension cause or promote keloid and hypertrophic scar pathogenesis? Wound Repair Regen. 2014;22(4):462–6.
8. Moustafa MF, Abdel-Fattah MA, Abdel-Fattah DC. Presumptive evidence of the effect of pregnancy estrogens on keloid growth. Case report. Plast Reconstr Surg. 1975;56(4):450–3.
9. Mendelsohn ME, Karas RH. Estrogen and the blood vessel wall. Curr Opin Cardiol. 1994;9(5):619–26.
10. Ogawa R, Okai K, Tokumura F, Mori K, Ohmori Y, Huang C, Hyakusoku H, Akaishi S. The relationship between skin stretching/contraction and pathologic scarring: the important role of mechanical forces in keloid generation. Wound Repair Regen. 2012;20(2):149–57.
11. Ogawa R, Akaishi S, Huang C, Dohi T, Aoki M, Omori Y, Koike S, Kobe K, Akimoto M, Hyakusoku H. Clinical applications of basic research that shows reducing skin tension could prevent and treat abnormal scarring: the importance of fascial/subcutaneous tensile reduction sutures and flap surgery for keloid and hypertrophic scar reconstruction. J Nippon Med Sch. 2011;78(2):68–76.
12. Akaishi S, Akimoto M, Ogawa R, Hyakusoku H. The relationship between keloid growth pattern and stretching tension: visual analysis using the finite element method. Ann Plast Surg. 2008;60(4):445–51.
13. Koike S, Akaishi S, Nagashima Y, Dohi T, Hyakusoku H, Ogawa R. Nd:YAG laser treatment for keloids and hypertrophic scars: an analysis of 102 cases. Plast Reconstr Surg Glob Open. 2015;2(12):e272.
14. Akaishi S, Koike S, Dohi T, Kobe K, Hyakusoku H, Ogawa R. Nd:YAG laser treatment of keloids and hypertrophic scars. Eplasty. 2012;12:e1.
15. Dover JS, Arndt KA. New approaches to the treatment of vascular lesions. Lasers Surg Med. 2000;26(2):158–63.
16. Alster TS, Williams C. Treatment of keloid sternotomy scars with 585 nm flashlamp-pumped pulsed-dye laser. Lancet. 1995;345:1198–200.
17. Paquet P, Hermanns JF, Pierard GE. Effect of the 585nm flash-pumped pulsed dye laser for the treatment of keloids. Dermatol Surg. 2001;27(2):171–4.
18. Dragoni F, Bassi A, Cannarozzo G, Bonan P, Moretti S, Campolmi P. Successful treatment of acne keloidalis nuchae resistant to conventional therapy with 1064-nm ND:YAG laser. G Ital Dermatol Venereol. 2013;148(2):231–2.
19. Rossi A, Lu R, Frey MK, Kubota T, Smith LA, Perez M. The use of the 300 microsecond 1064 nm Nd:YAG laser in the treatment of keloids. J Drugs Dermatol. 2013;12(11):1256–62.
20. Al-Mohamady AE, Ibrahim SM, Muhammad MM. Pulsed dye laser versus long-pulsed Nd:YAG laser in the treatment of hypertrophic scars and keloid: a comparative randomized split-scar trial. J Cosmet Laser Ther. 2016;8:1–5.
21. Tian WC. Savior of post-blepharoepicanthoplasty scarring: novel use of a low-fluence 1064-nm Q-switched Nd:YAG laser. J Cosmet Laser Ther. 2016;18(2):69–71.

Intense Pulsed Light (IPL) Monotherapy for Scars

Umarah Muhammad, Yvonne Stubbington,
and Kayvan Shokrollahi

1 Background

Intense pulsed light (IPL) is a non-coherent filtered flash lamp, emitting a broadband spectrum (515–1200 nm) of visible polychromatic-pulsed light of a high intensity [1]. As such, it is not a laser technology per se using a filter to narrow the spectrum of light rather than emitting a single wavelength of light as lasers do. Its use was first conceived as therapeutic treatment of vascular lesions in 1992 [2].

IPL has largely evolved over time, from single pulse systems to multiple sequential pulsing, with the ability to use different cut off wavelengths, spectral output and size of delivered light [2]. This makes the grouping of IPL studies challenging. Its efficacy has been recently reported in the treatment of photo-damaged facial skin, promoting the production of neo collagen and ordering of elastic fibres [1].

The wide range of wavelengths has made it a versatile tool with a well-recognised role in the treatment of the following conditions: photo-damaged skin [3], hyperpigmentation disorders [4], cutaneous vascular malformations [5], telangiectasia [6], photo-epilation [7], lentigines [8], tattoo elimination [5], acne and hair removal [9], as well as a method of non-ablative skin rejuvenation to remodel skin collagen [10].

A systematic review of IPL in the management of various dermatological disorders found level 1 evidence for the use of IPL in managing conditions such as melasma, acne vulgaris and telangiectasia [2]. However, with regard to hypertrophic and keloid scars, there was a much weaker level of evidence (defined as the highest level of evidence being limited to open level trials with the controls having no treatment). The conclusion of the review was that multiple sessions of IPL may be effective for the treatment of scars but less so for atrophic variants [2], although it is important to note that these conclusions were based on the results of only five studies on hypertrophic and keloid scars [2].

2 Keloid and Hypertrophic Scarring

Keloid and hypertrophic scars result from an abnormal wound healing process, which includes excessive proliferation of fibroblasts, a prolonged phase of inflammation and fibroplasias combined with increased collagen synthesis, although their accurate pathogenesis remains unknown [11, 12]. The key characteristics to their appearance clinically include: a papule or plaque scar which is erythematous or purple in colour, firm to touch, with a well-demarcated edge occasionally associated with pain and pruritis [13].

Treatment modalities range from topical and intra-lesional steroids (the current gold standard) [14] to cryotherapy, radiation, surgical excision and pressure dressings; however, no single method of treatment is without its limitations [15–17].

3 The Use of IPL Alone

A case series by Piccolo et al. investigated the efficacy of IPL in 58 unconventional cases including five hypertrophic scars and five keloid scars with the remaining cases ranging from rosacea and port wine stains to sarcoidosis. Dermatoscopic images demonstrated a significant reduction of the vascular component in the thicker areas, with most scars flattened and smaller after three sessions. No two patients in this series were treated with the same settings in terms of filters, number of pulses/pulse duration and fluences. This highlights two important aspects with regard to using IPL: firstly, where the therapeutic effect lies with IPL is difficult to establish as there is often no consistency in the types of settings used in studies. In contrast, the adjustability of such settings allows

U. Muhammad · Y. Stubbington
Mersey Regional Centre for Burns and Plastic Surgery, Whiston Hospital, Liverpool, UK
e-mail: yvonne.stubbington@sthk.nhs.uk

K. Shokrollahi (✉)
Burns and Plastic Surgery Unit, Whiston Hospital, Liverpool, UK

K. Shokrollahi (ed.), *Laser Management of Scars*, https://doi.org/10.1007/978-3-030-52919-2_8

for the tailoring and personalisation of IPL in accordance with the patient needs. Authors concluded that IPL could represent a valid therapeutic option as it provides excellent outcomes, flexibility in treatment with a low side effect profile [9].

Sarkar et al. investigated the use of IPL on immature burn scars, which had healed within 2 months using conservative measures. Nineteen patients each had four treatment sessions. Authors found vascularity, pliability and height significantly improved when assessed using the Vancouver scar scale. Authors concluded IPL was a well-tolerated treatment modality in this cohort of patients [10].

A case report of 3 patients with hypertrophic scarring treated with IPL found a definite improvement in scar tissue appearance. IPL with the correct outputs was concluded to be an effective tool for treatment of inflamed hypertrophic and colloidal scars. The main filters used in these three cases were 515, 550, 590 and 610 nm [18].

4 IPL Treatment Combined with Intra-Lesional Steroids

A clinical trial, which compared outcomes using the Vancouver scar scale of 166 keloid and hypertrophic scars treated with cryotherapy (control group) to IPL (treatment group) found both the recovery and complication rates to be higher in the control group. Both groups also received intralesional steroids. The scars completely cured were 166, 83 of these scars were treated by IPL and 83 by cryotherapy. The most common complication reported equally in both patient groups was hyperpigmentation. Both methods produced high levels of patient satisfaction with a percentage cure rate of 80.7% for cryotherapy and 73.5% for IPL [19]. This study provides a perfect example as to how IPL is often studied in conjunction with alternative modalities, which furthers the challenge for researchers when attempting to compare the outcomes of a particular intervention.

Kim et al. conducted a pilot study of 58 patients with keloid and hypertrophic scars treated with a combination of IPL and intra-lesional corticosteroids at 4–8-week treatment intervals. The stratum corneum (SC) barrier function was also measured for 12 patients using transepidermal water loss (TEWL) and SC capacitance. Outcomes were assessed using the modified Vancouver scar scale, physician's global assessment and patient satisfaction score. This pilot study demonstrated a significant clinical improvement in all three scores with combined IPL and corticosteroid treatment, with a significant decrease of TEWL and elevation of SC capacitance. Authors concluded this method of combined treatment improves both scar appearance and recovery level of skin hydration status in terms of skin barrier function [13].

5 IPL Treatment Combined with CO_2 Laser

Wang et al. evaluated the effect of IPL combined with CO_2 laser on acne scarring in 37 Chinese patients. Patients underwent 4–6 sessions of IPL followed by two sessions of carbon dioxide laser. Outcomes were evaluated using dermatologist assessment of skin colour (erythema index and melanin index), sebum secretion and skin hydration as well as patient self-assessment. Treatment with IPL alone reduced both the inflammatory lesion and atrophic scar scores. Further treatment with CO_2 laser further reduced the atrophic scar scores. Both scores remained low at a 6-month follow-up with 90% of patients reporting significant or moderate overall improvement. This combination of lasers was concluded to be effective in patients with both atrophic and inflammatory acne scarring with an acceptable adverse effect profile [20].

6 IPL vs. Other Treatment Modalities

Erol et al. conducted a prospective cohort study of 109 patients with hypertrophic scars and keloids as a result of burns, trauma, surgery or acne [21]. Scars were treated with IPL Quantum TM2, with 2–4-week intervals between an average of eight treatments. The scar appearance was assessed by two physicians blinded to study patients and treatments. Photographs of the scars were graded 0–4 for clinical improvement in reduction in height, erythema and hardness. The percentage of the patients in the study who had overall clinical improvement was 92.5, this was defined as excellent in 31.2%, good in 25.7%, moderate in 34% and minimal in 9.1% [21]. This study was novel as it also assessed the preventative role of IPL. Sixty-five percent of the 17 patients with a known predisposition to hypertrophic scarring had good-excellent improvement in the resultant scarring with the use of IPL in a preventative capacity. Authors concluded that IPL was effective in improving appearance of keloid/hypertrophic scar irrespective of origin, as it noticeably reduced height, redness and hardness [21]. The authors correctly recognise that the use of the IPL in the prevention of surgical scar formation has not been adequately assessed [21]. There are several unanswered questions in this regard including: how soon postoperatively could IPL be used postoperatively to prevent hypertrophic scar formation? Could this be as soon as suture removal, or would this have adverse implications for wound healing? Additionally how do we determine which patients would benefit most from such intervention? and how do we know that the patient would not develop a scar irrespective of preventative treatment? [21].

Bellew et al. conducted a prospective cohort study which compared outcomes between two groups with hypertrophic surgical scars (from breast reduction or abdominoplasty) treated with either IPL or 595-nm long-pulsed dye laser (LPDL) [22]. Patients had two treatments, which were 2 months apart. Physician global assessment scores of improvement were used to assess outcomes with side-by-side comparison of pre- and post-operative photographs. Authors also assessed patient pain scores and the presence of post-treatment purpura. The mean improvement on a 0 to 3-point scale was 2.2 (55%) after the first LPDL treatment and 3.2 (80%) after the second. Mean improvement was 1.8 (45%) after the first IPL treatment and 2.6 (65%) after the second, although these differences between the two treatment modalities were not statistically significant. Patients rated IPL as more painful than LPDL, although the incidence of post-treatment purpura was lower with IPL. Authors concluded that LPDL and IPL were equally as effective in improving the appearance of hypertrophic surgical scars, with IPL minimising the risk of purpura [22]. Many authors fail to comment on the size and height of scars and if these were similar between individuals studied, significant variation between the scar height and size between intervention groups may present as a confounding variable when attempting to establish the true benefit of IPL vs. other treatment modalities.

7 Complications Reported with IPL

IPL is generally well tolerated with minimal risks associated with its use and is regarded to have a "benign side effect profile", with commonly cited adverse effects in the literature including mild discomfort, erythema, purpura, oedema, blistering and crusting which typically last up to 48 h [2]. However, some studies have reported further complications with its use. A cohort study, which looked into the side effects of IPL when used for hair removal, noted some cases of post-inflammatory hyperpigmentation (n = 75), post-inflammatory hypopigmentation (n = 10), bullae formation (n = 64) and scar formation (n = 1). Leukotrichia, folliculitis and paradoxical hypertrichosis were also noted in smaller numbers of patients [23]. In a prospective cohort study assessing the benefit of IPL for post-burn hyperpigmentation, 3 of 19 patients developed blisters and 1 patient erythema which all subsequently resolved in 1 week without any permanent scarring [24]. Ozdemir et al. reported two cases of blistering which lead to hypertrophic scarring with the use of IPL in the treatment of facial port wine stains [25].

8 Conclusion

The unique selling point of IPL over other treatment modalities remains its wide range of wavelengths alongside the adjustability of settings, which allows for personalisation of the treatment for the patient.

Although IPL may have a role in the management of hypertrophic and keloid scars, a major limitation of the existing evidence base is the lack of rigorous study design and controls with the majority of data being limited to uncontrolled, open-label trials and retrospective studies. It becomes challenging for clinicians to compare the efficacy of IPL across studies as IPL is often studied in conjunction with intra-lesional steroids [13] or with additional methods of laser treatment [20]. Important unanswered questions within the published literature on IPL for the management of hypertrophic and keloid scars include:

- Is there an optimal combination of settings (filters, number of pulses/pulse duration and fluences), which holds superiority over another?
- The role of IPL in the prevention of hypertrophic scar formation and how soon post-operatively could we laser?
- Does the true benefit of IPL lie in combination with more established methods of treatment such as intra-lesional steroids or other lasers?
- A more in-depth and robust side effect profile, based on studies with larger sample sizes with longer periods of follow up is warranted.

References

1. Hernádez-Pérez E, Colombo-Charrier E, Valencia-Ibiett E. Intense pulsed light in the treatment of striae distensae. Dermatol Surg. 2002;28(12):1124–30. [cited 2018 Jun 28];28(2):1124–30. https://doi.org/10.1046/j.1524-4725.2002.02111.x.
2. Wat H, Wu DC, Rao J, Goldman MP. Application of intense pulsed light in the treatment of dermatologic disease: a systematic review. Dermatol Surg. 2014;40(4):359–77. [cited 2018 Jun 28]. https://doi.org/10.1111/dsu.12424.
3. Varughese N, Goldberg D, Keller L. Split face comparison between single-band and dual band pulsed light technology for treatment of photodamage. J Cosmet Laser Ther. 2016;18(4):213–6. https://doi.org/10.1080/14764172.2016.1177188.
4. Hultman CS, Friedstat JS, Edkins RE. Efficacy of intense pulsed light for the treatment of burn scar dyschromias: a pilot study to assess patient satisfaction, safety, and willingness to pay. Ann Plast Surg. 2015;74(Suppl 4):S204–8. https://doi.org/10.1097/SAP.0000000000000447.
5. Raulin C, Schroeter CA, Weiss RA, Keiner M, Werner S. Treatment of port-wine stains with a noncoherent pulsed light source: a retrospective study. Arch Dermatol. 1999;135(6):679–83. [cited 2019 Mar 24]. https://doi.org/10.1001/archderm.135.6.679.
6. Raulin C, Weiss RA, Schönermark MP. Treatment of essential telangiectasias with an intense pulsed light source (PhotoDerm VL). Dermatol Surg. 1997;23(10):941–5. [cited 2019 Mar 24]. https://doi.org/10.1111/j.1524-4725.1997.tb00755.x.
7. Sadick NS, Weiss RA, Shea CR, Nagel H, Nicholson J, Prieto VG. Long-term photoepilation using a broad-spectrum intense pulsed light source. Arch Dermatol. 2000;136(11):1336–40. [cited 2019 Mar 24]. https://doi.org/10.1001/archderm.136.11.1336.
8. Raulin C, Goldman MP, Weiss MA, Weiss RA. Treatment of adult port-wine stains using intense pulsed light therapy (PhotoDerm VL): brief initial clinical report. Dermatol Surg. 1997;23(7):594–7.

[cited 2019 Mar 24]. https://doi.org/10.1111/j.1524-4725.1997.tb00698.x.
9. Piccolo D, Di Marcantonio D, Crisman G, Cannarozzo G, Sannino M, Chiricozzi A, et al. Unconventional use of intense pulsed light. Biomed Res Int. 2014;2014:618206. [cited 2018 Sep 10]. Available from: http://www.hindawi.com/journals/bmri/2014/618206/.
10. Sarkar A, Dewangan YK, Bain J, Rakshit P, Dhruw K, Basu SK, et al. Effect of intense pulsed light on immature burn scars: a clinical study. Indian J Plast Surg. 2014;47(3):381–5. https://doi.org/10.4103/2F0970-0358.146596.
11. Alster T, West T. Treatment of scars: a review. Ann Plast Surg. 1997;39(4):418–32. Available from https://journals.lww.com/annalsplasticsurgery/Abstract/1997/10000/Treatment_of_Scars__A_Review.14.aspx.
12. English R, Shenefelt P. Keloids and hypertrophic scars. Dermatol Surg. 1999;25(8):631–8. https://doi.org/10.1046/j.1524-4725.1999.98257.x.
13. Kim DY, Park HS, Yoon HS, Cho S. Efficacy of IPL device combined with intralesional corticosteroid injection for the treatment of keloids and hypertrophic scars with regards to the recovery of skin barrier function: a pilot study. J Dermatolog Treat. 2015;26(5):481–4. [cited 2018 Sep 10]. https://doi.org/10.3109/09546634.2015.1024598.
14. Leventhal D, Furr M, Reiter D. Treatment of keloids and hypertrophic scars: a meta-analysis and review of the literature. Arch Facial Plast Surg. 2006;8(6):362–8. https://doi.org/10.1001/archfaci.8.6.362.
15. Mamalis A, Lev-Tov H, Nguyen D, Jagdeo JR. Laser and light based treatment of keloids - a review. J Eur Acad Dermatol. 2014;28(6):689–99. https://doi.org/10.1111/jdv.12253.
16. Arno AI, Gauglitz GG, Barret JP, Jeschke MG. Up to date approach to manage keloids and hypertrophic scars: a useful guide. Burns. 2014;40(7):1255–66. https://doi.org/10.1016/j.burns.2014.02.011.
17. Durani P, Bayat A. Levels of evidence for the treatment of keloid disease. J Plast Reconstr Aesthet Surg. 2008;61(1):4–17. https://doi.org/10.1016/j.bjps.2007.05.007.
18. Cartier H. Use of intense pulsed light in the treatment of scars. J Cosmet Dermatol. 2005;4(1):34–40. [cited 2018 Sep 10]. https://doi.org/10.1111/j.1473-2165.2005.00157.x.
19. Meymandi SS, Moosazadeh M, Rezazadeh A. Comparing two methods of cryotherapy and intense pulsed light with triamcinolone injection in the treatment of keloid and hypertrophic scars: a clinical trial. Osong public Heal Res Perspect. 2016;7(5):313–9. [cited 2018 Sep 10]. https://doi.org/10.1016/2Fj.phrp.2016.08.005.
20. Wang B, Wu Y, Luo YJ, Xu XG, Xu TH, Chen JZ, et al. Combination of intense pulsed light and fractional CO(2) laser treatments for patients with acne with inflammatory and scarring lesions. Clin Exp Dermatol. 2013;38(4):344–51. https://doi.org/10.1111/ced.12010.
21. Erol OO, Gurlek A, Agaoglu G, Topcuoglu E, Oz H. Treatment of hypertrophic scars and keloids using intense pulsed light (IPL). Aesthetic Plast Surg. 2008;32(6):902–9. [cited 2018 Sep 10]. https://doi.org/10.1007/s00266-008-9161-7.
22. Bellew SG, Weiss MA, Weiss RA. Comparison of intense pulsed light to 595-nm long-pulsed pulsed dye laser for treatment of hypertrophic surgical scars: a pilot study. J Drugs Dermatol. 2005;4(4):448–52. [cited 2018 Sep 10] Available from: http://www.ncbi.nlm.nih.gov/pubmed/16004017.
23. Radmanesh M, Azar-Beig M, Abtahian A, Naderi AH. Burning, paradoxical hypertrichosis, leukotrichia and folliculitis are four major complications of intense pulsed light hair removal therapy. J Dermatol Treat. 2008;19(6):360–3. https://doi.org/10.1080/09546630802132627.
24. Ho WS, Chan HH, Ying SY, Chan PC, Burd A, King WW. Prospective study on the treatment of postburn hyperpigmentation by intense pulsed light. Lasers Surg Med. 2003;32(1):42–5. https://doi.org/10.1002/lsm.10139.
25. Ozdemir M, Engin B, Mevlitoglu I. Treatment of facial port-wine stains with intense pulsed light: a prospective study. J Cosmet Dermatol. 2008;7(2):127–31. https://doi.org/10.1111/j.1473-2165.2008.00375.x.

Nd:YAG Laser and Intense Pulsed Light (IPL) in the Treatment of Hypertrophic and Keloid Scar

Jared L. Potts, Jillian M. McLaughlin, Dexter W. Weeks, Ludwik K. Branski, and William B. Norbury

M22™ is a modular multi-application platform (Lumenis, Santa Clara, CA) that combines universal intense pulsed light (IPL), multi-spot Nd:YAG, ResurFX™, and Q-switched Nd:YAG. The Nd:YAG and intense pulsed light components of the M22™ have been utilized in the treatment of hypertrophic scars and keloids. M22™ is utilized at Shriners Hospital for Children in Galveston, using the intense pulse light function, for the treatment of immature and pruritic hypertrophic burn scars. A picture of the M22™ utilized at Shriners Hospital for Children in Galveston can be seen in Fig. 1. Its use as well as the use of intense pulsed light and Nd:YAG in the treatment of hypertrophic burn scars and keloids as described in the literature will be reviewed in detail in this chapter.

1 Introduction

Historically, vascular-specific, flashlamp-pumped 585- and 595-nm pulsed dye laser were used for vascular malformations by selectively targeting its chromophore hemoglobin. Limitations of pulse dye lasers include a very short pulse duration (0.45 ms) and shallow penetrating wavelength (585 nm), therefore making it only effective in treating superficial vessels. Additionally, PDL works by *coagulating the microvasculature*, breaking it abruptly apart and as a side effect can produce long-lasting purpura [1]. As an alternative to PDL, IPL and Nd:YAG have been used in the treatment of vascular malformations, hypertrophic, and keloid scar.

First introduced in 1990s, intense pulsed light (IPL) was initially described and utilized for the treatment of lower-limb telangiectasias. Although not technically a laser, IPL delivers a focused and controlled light energy. Light pulses are generated by a burst of electrical current passing through a xenon lamp onto the skin via a conduction crystal within a

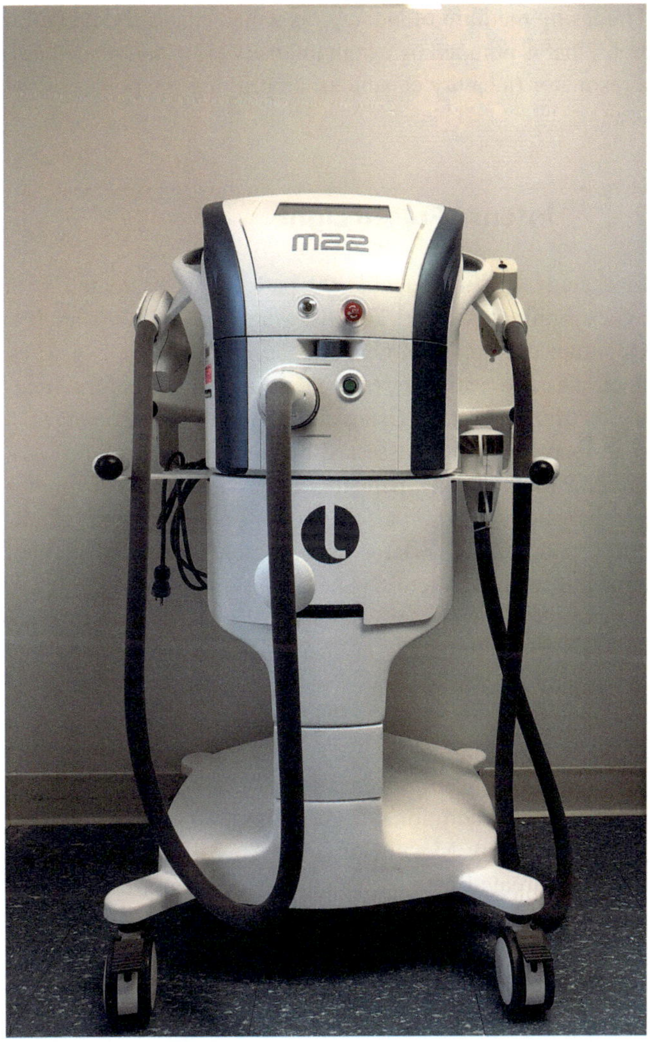

Fig. 1 M22™ platform utilized at Shriners Hospital for Children in Galveston

J. L. Potts · J. M. McLaughlin · D. W. Weeks · L. K. Branski
W. B. Norbury (✉)
Division of Plastic Surgery, Department of Surgery, The University of Texas Medical Branch, Shriners Hospital for Children, Galveston, TX, USA
e-mail: jalpotts@utmb.edu; jmmclaug@utmb.edu; dwweeks@utmb.edu; lubransk@utmb.edu; wbnorbur@utmb.edu

K. Shokrollahi (ed.), *Laser Management of Scars*, https://doi.org/10.1007/978-3-030-52919-2_9

handpiece. The pulsed light is polychromatic, non-coherent, and broad-spectrum in the wavelength range between 390 and 1200 nm, allowing various chromophores, such as hemoglobin, water, and melanin, to be targeted. Through the use of specific filters, IPL can selectively target desired cellular or structural elements leading to its wide variety of uses including treatment of vascular malformations, pigmented lesions, and hair removal [2].

First introduced in the 1960s, Nd:YAG, Neodymium-doped Yttrium-Aluminum-Garnet, was the first laser to be used clinically in the treatment of massive gastrointestinal bleeding. It is a solid-state laser capable of producing a near-infrared wavelength that penetrates deep into the skin and is readily absorbed by hemoglobin and melanin chromophores. The lasing medium of Nd:YAG is a man-made crystal (solid state) that is pumped by a high intensity lamp and placed into a resonator (a cavity capable of amplifying the power of the laser).

2 Intense Pulsed Light

In a study by Erol et al., 109 patients were treated with hypertrophic scars and keloids were treated using an IPL Quantum device. Treatment was administered at 2–4-week intervals, and patients received an average of eight treatments (range = 6–24). Using digital photographs, changes in scar appearance were assessed by two physicians who were blinded to the study patients and treatments. The photographs were graded on a scale of 0–4 (none, minimal, moderate, good, excellent) for improvement in overall clinical appearance and reduction in height, erythema, and hardness. An overall clinical improvement in the appearance of scars and reductions in height, erythema, and hardness were seen in the majority of the patients (92.5%). Improvement was excellent in 31.2% of the patients, good in 25.7%, moderate in 34%, and minimal in 9.1%. Over half the patients had good or excellent improvement [3]. Similar positive results are seen in two additional studies [4, 5].

In a study by Meymandi et al., 86 patients with keloid scar were treated with a combination of intense pulsed light plus intralesional corticosteroid. The level of clinical improvement, color improvement and scar height was 89.1%, 88.8%, and 89.1%, respectively. The incidence of complications (1 telangiectasia case, 7 hyperpigmentation cases and 2 atrophy cases) following treatment with IPL was 11.6%. Moreover, the participants' satisfaction with IPL method was 88.8%. Another study also found similar findings in 52 patients treated with IPL and intralesional corticosteroid, along with a decrease in transepidermal water loss, indicating that hypertrophic scars and keloids treated with IPL and intralesional corticosteroid were becoming more similar to that of normal unscarred skin [6].

3 Nd:YAG

In a study by Akaishi et al., 6 patients with hypertrophic scars and 16 patients with keloid were treated with long-pulsed, 1064-nm Nd:YAG in noncontact mode with low fluence and a submillisecond pulse duration [7]. Patients underwent an average of eight treatments and scar scores were analyzed pre- and posttreatment. All patients had a decrease in scar scale score; however, this did not reach statistical significance. In a follow-up study by the same group, 38 patients with hypertrophic scars and 64 patients with keloid scar were treated with long-pulsed 1064-nm Nd:YAG. Patients underwent an average of 6–12 sessions depending on the anatomical site. All patients had a significant decrease in the pre- versus posttreatment scar scale scores; however, 1 patient experienced a recurrence of hypertrophic scar at 6 months and 42% of patients experienced recurrence of keloid scar at 6 months [8]. Additional studies on the use of long-pulsed 1064-nm Nd:YAG in the treatment of keloids showed variable rates of efficacy, with all the articles reporting a decrease in scar thickness and complete resolution of keloid in 10–60% of patients and partial resolution of keloid in 41–63% of patients [9–15]. Adjuvant intralesional 5-fluorouracil and/or intralesional corticosteroid was also found to be more effective than Nd:YAG alone [15].

Studies comparing Nd:YAG to PDL have found Nd:YAG to be equally effective or more effective than PDL in the treatment of hypertrophic scars [16, 17]. Complications following PDL and Nd:YAG are comparable, with conflicting reports of which modality produces more pain [13, 18].

4 Treatment Methodology/Regimen

Similar to that described by Hultman et al., our approach is to use laser or intense pulsed light in a defined sequence, to address specific pathological components of the hypertrophic burn scar and keloid [19]. In our practice at Shriners Hospital for Children in Galveston, we have found that intense pulsed light is more effective in reducing the hyperemia and edema of the immature burn scars and has led to a significant decrease in associated burn scar pruritus. The Itch Man Scale is a previously validated and reliable tool to assess itching in pediatric burn patients and helps to quantify post-burn pruritus [20]. A decrease in pre- and posttreatment Itch Man scale scores has been observed in patients treated with intense pulse light.

Intense pulse light has replaced the use of pulsed dye laser at our institution for early scar management, while ablative, fractional, 10,600-nm wavelength CO_2 laser resurfacing is used to correct abnormal texture, thickness, and stiffness of the more mature scar.

Table 1 Intense Pulsed Light and Nd:YAG Laser recommended settings for hypertrophic scar or keloid

Intense Pulsed Light (Lumenis M-22™; Lumenis, Santa Clara, CA, USA)	
Wavelength filter	590 nm
Single/double/triple pulse	Triple pulse
Pulse duration	5 ms
Delay	20 ms
Fluence	15–27 J/cm^2
Guide	Large rectangular light guide
Requires	Optical coupling gel
Nd:YAG Laser (Cutera®, Brisbane, California)	
Wavelength	1064 nm
Spot size	5 mm
Pulse duration	0.25 ms
Cooling	Yes, via copper-cooling tip
Energy density	65–75 J/cm^2
Repetition rate	2 Hz
Overlap	No
End point	3 passes or if pain experienced following second pass

Common Intense Pulsed Light and Nd:YAG Laser Settings for Hypertrophic Scar or Keloid. Nd:YAG Laser settings adapted from Koike et al. [8]. Please note that these settings are suggestions based on current literature and clinical experience. These settings can and should be modified in accordance to patient factors (e.g., tolerance of treatment or treatment response), developing technologies, and/or machine or factory specific model recommendations/settings

The treatment settings for the intense pulse light (Lumenis M22™ Santa Clara, CA) are reviewed in Table 1, and the standard laser log utilized at our institution is seen in Fig. 2.

Patients are asked to wash with chlorhexidine soap the night prior to the procedure. Depending on the age of the patient, general or topical anesthetic is administered. A coupling gel is applied topically to the skin prior to the use of the intense pulsed light device to minimize damage to the epidermis. Following treatment, a soothing aloe vera cream, a gentle cleansing soap, and a sunscreen (SPF 50 or above) are prescribed to each patient after each session. Patients generally do not require postoperative analgesics for pain and, if necessary, are provided with acetaminophen and/or ibuprofen depending on patient preference and/or tolerance.

Multiple factors are taken into account in order to determine patient's treatment regimen including: results following initial intense pulsed light treatment, severity of burn scar pruritus, and continued presence of immature scar. There is no limit to the number of treatments provided to patients, and treatments are provided to patients at 20–30-day intervals.

Although, Nd:YAG is not utilized in our institution for the management of hypertrophic scars or keloids. For completeness, the typical treatment settings obtained from the largest series utilizing long-pulsed 1064-nm Nd:YAG for hypertrophic scar and keloid are reviewed in Table 1.

Utilizing our experience in treating vascular malformations with Nd:YAG, both the pre- and postoperative management parallels that of intense pulsed light with one exception, due to increased pain associated with Nd:YAG use, our pediatric patient's more often opt to undergo general anesthesia prior to Nd:YAG treatment.

5 Clinical Examples

Shriners Hospital for Children in Galveston first began utilizing M22™ platform in 2016. Since that time, 56 patients have undergone treatment with the intense pulsed light modality for treatment of immature, pruritic hypertrophic burn scars. Patients receive an average of three treatments spaced 1 month apart (range: 1–8 treatments). Clinical examples of patients more than 1-year posttreatment will be reviewed.

Patient 1 is a 6-year-old male with a history of 72% TBSA flame burn (64% third degree TBSA) involving the anterior and posterior trunk, bilateral upper, and lower extremities. Patient had severely pruritic immature hypertrophic burn scars involving the posterior trunk. Despite routine management for control of burn scar pruritus, patient continued to have severe pruritus which often led to the development of excoriated skin and unhealed open wounds. Patient 1 underwent a total of four treatments each spaced an average of 1–2 months apart. Itch Man Scale Scores decreased from 4 at the initial IPL treatment to 1 following the last IPL treatment. Photos of patient's clinical course are seen in Figs. 3, 4, and 5.

Patient 2 is an 8-year-old female with a history of a 38% TBSA flame burn (22% third degree) involving the face, bilateral upper, and lower extremities. Patient had severely pruritus and immature hypertrophic burn scars along bilateral cheeks and nose, despite conservative management. Patient underwent a total of two treatments to the bilateral cheeks and nose spaced 1 month apart. Itch Man Scale Scores decreased from 4 at the initial IPL treatment to 2 following the last IPL treatment. Photos of patient's clinical course are seen in Figs. 6 and 7.

6 Discussion

Due to comparatively longer wavelengths, both IPL and Nd:YAG can penetrate deeper within the tissue affecting more deeply located vessels and dermal components than PDL [6, 21]. Comparatively to PDL, modern IPL devices and long-pulsed Nd:YAG can provide longer pulse durations, which, depending on the device, can be as high as 100 ms. This longer pulse duration enables delivery of energy to vessels over longer periods of time, resulting in

Shriners Hospitals for Children®

M22-Nd:YAG

LASER Treatment Compliance Checklist

Serial No. 20014

Patient Sticker

Treatment No. _____

Skin Type: I II III IV V VI	Procedure:	No. of pulses since last calibration:
Skin condition to be tested:______		Test Patch:______
Size: ______ Colour: ______	Density: ______	Texture: ______ Depth: ______

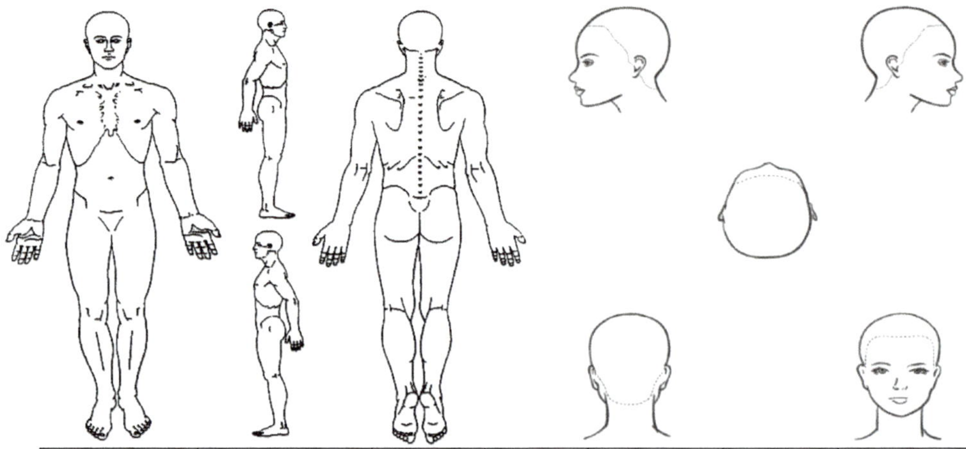

HP (IPL/Nd:YAG)	Spot Size (Large/Small)	Filter	Pulse (1,2,3)	PW [ms]	D [ms]	Fμ/cm2	Cooling (On/Off)	Number of Pulses

Preoperative:

- ☐ Key Retrieved designated area
- ☐ Laser Door Signs/Goggle posted
- ☐ Windows covered
- ☐ Appropriate eyewear examined
- ☐ Laser equipment examined
- ☐ Water/Saline on back field
- ☐ Non-Reflective basin
- ☐ Sterile Scalpel/Hemostats available on back field
- ☐ Fire extinguisher available

Intraoperative:

- ☐ Authorized personnel only
- ☐ All persons in LTC wearing laser protective eyewear and PPE
- ☐ Patients eyes protected
- ☐ Treatment area thoroughly cleansed
- ☐ Laser Treatment Site:
    - o Hair closely shaved
    - o Clear Aquasonic Gel
- ☐ Wet Pack
    - o Nose/Mouth
    - o Rectum
- ☐ Non-*Reflective instruments utilized
- ☐ OR doors closed during laser activation
- ☐ Emergent airway supplies available

Postoperative:

- ☐ Laser documentation completed
- ☐ Laser console, hand pieces and accessories cleaned appropriately
- ☐ Laser console, hand pieces and accessories stored appropriately and returned without incident and in good condition
- ☐ Key returned to designated location

______________________ **RN**

Laser User (Physician): ______________________

Date: ______________________

Laser Operator (Tech/RN): ______________________

Fig. 2 Shriners Hospital for Children in Galveston Standard Laser Log Form

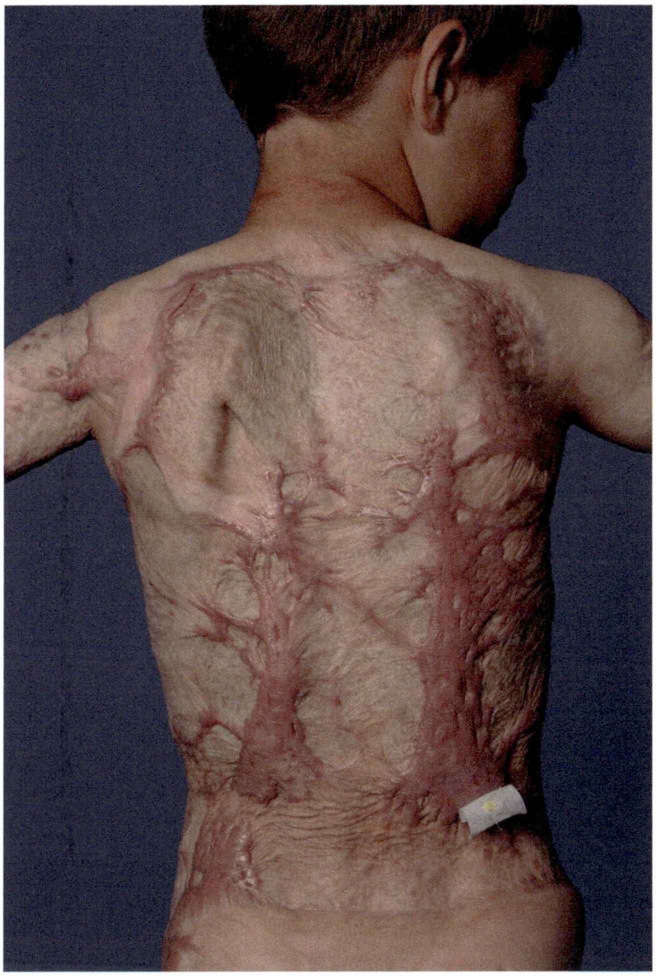

Fig. 3 Patient 1 is 13 months post-burn and is scheduled to undergo his first IPL treatment

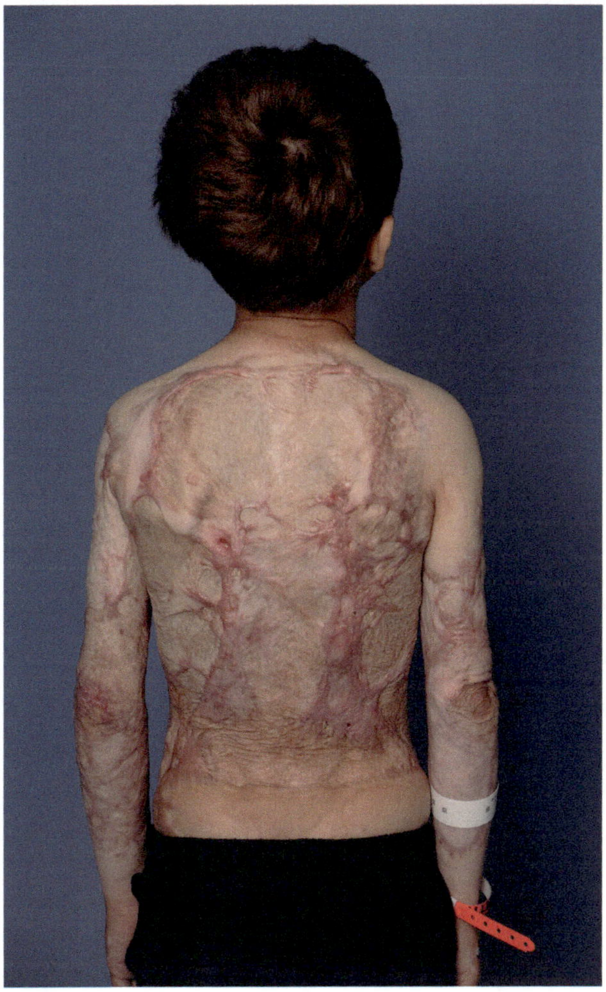

Fig. 4 Patient 1 is 19 months post-burn and has undergone two IPL treatments

gentle, uniform heating which reduces the chance of vessel rupture and posttreatment purpura. Compared to that of Nd:YAG and PDL, IPL has a larger spot size which allows for a larger area to be treated with each pulse. In the appropriate anatomical area this can lead to increased efficiency and decreased operative costs.

Similar to vascular malformations, hypertrophic scars and keloids contain an abnormal proliferation of blood vessels which likely contribute to abnormal collagen overgrowth. Suppression of these vessels in hypertrophic scar and keloid by pulsed dye laser has led to a decrease in scar height, erythema, scar-related pruritus, and an improvement in scar texture in both immature and mature scars [22]. As described by Hultman et al., laser or intense pulsed light should be used in a defined sequence, to address specific pathological components of the hypertrophic burn scar and keloid [19]. Hultman et al. describes using PDL to reduce hyperemia and edema of the immature burn scars. However, given the benefits of intense pulsed light as described above, IPL has replaced PDL for the treatment of immature, hyperemic burn scars at the Shriners Hospital for Galveston. For more mature hypertrophic burn scars, ablative fractional lasers (Erbium, CO_2) have become the gold standard. At Shriners Hospital for Galveston, it is standard to use ablative fractional 10,600-nm

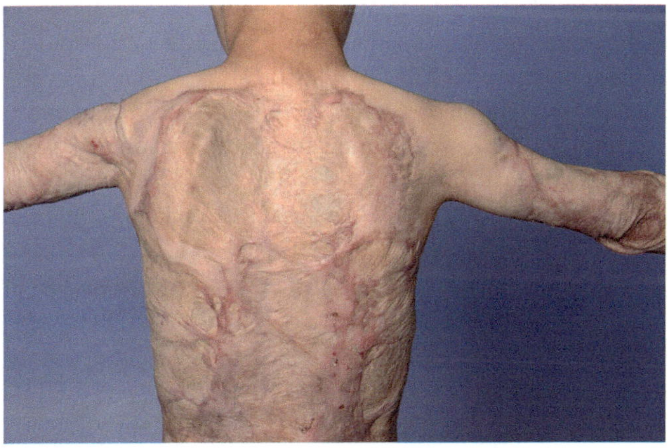

Fig. 5 Patient 1 is 25 months post-burn and has undergone four IPL treatments. Photos were taken 5 months following final IPL treatment and 1 year following initial IPL treatment

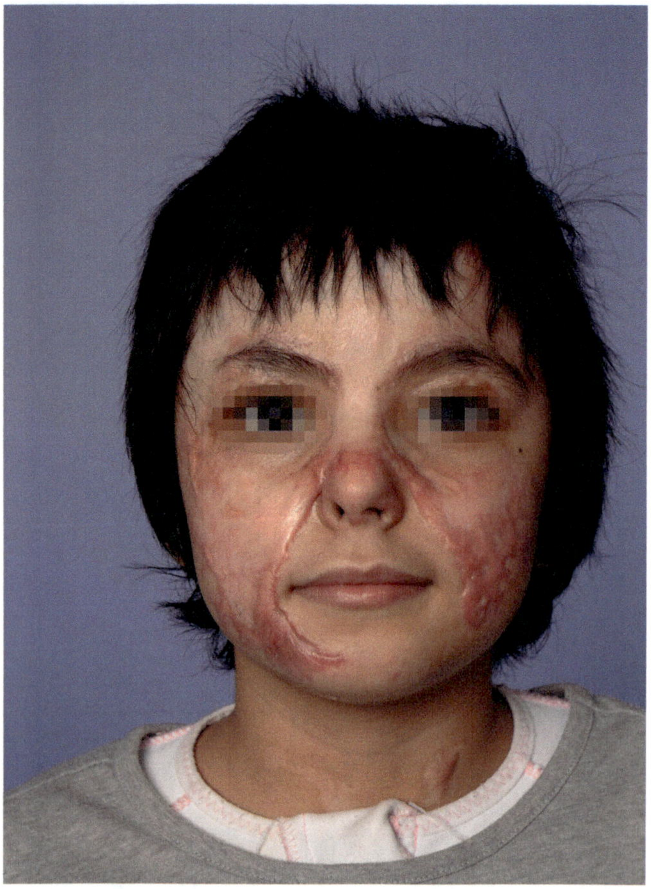

Fig. 6 Patient 2 is 6 months post-burn and is scheduled to undergo her first IPL treatment

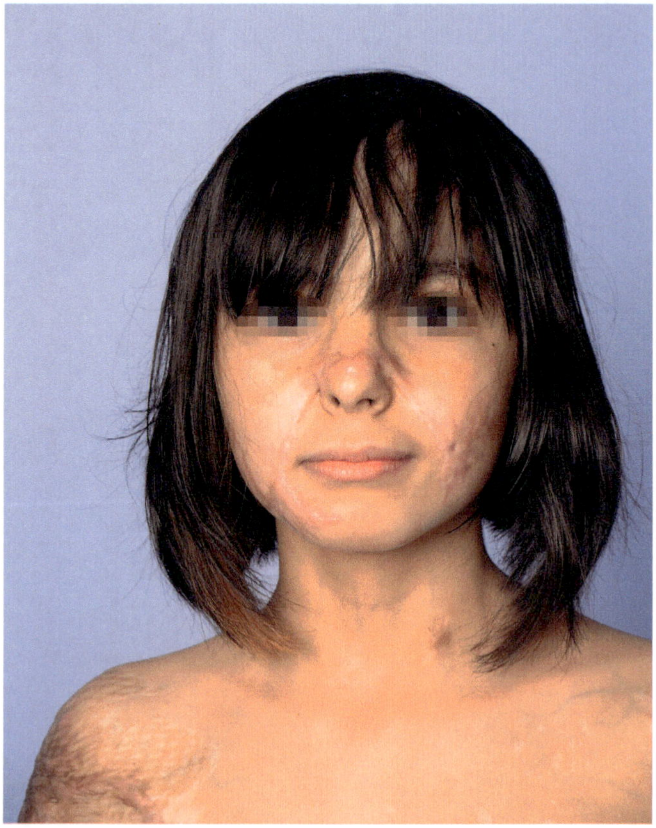

Fig. 7 Patient 2 is 18 months post-burn and has undergone two IPL treatments. Photos were taken 11 months following final IPL treatment and 1 year following initial IPL treatment

CO_2 laser which targets the chromophore water in collagen. The vaporization of this water results in the fragmentation and removal of scar, to create a pore within the scar tissue up to 4 mm in depth, surrounding which is an area of thermocoagulation. These two result in modulation of the abnormal scar and production of new collagen in a controlled manner.

Both Nd:YAG, as a non-ablative non fractionated laser, and IPL create a controlled thermal injury to the dermis that initiate a cascade of wound healing and remodeling events, resulting in neocollagenesis. However, both Nd:YAG and intense pulsed light are far less efficacious in collagen remodeling than the gold standard, fractional ablative lasers (Erbium, CO_2). Advantages of Nd:YAG and intense pulsed light over fractional ablative lasers include less downtime and less pain; however, multiple treatments are often necessary to achieve results comparable to that of fractional ablative lasers, i.e., 10,600-nm CO_2 laser, which can lead to higher costs. However, this laser is not the primary laser used by the authors for treatment of hypertrophic or keloid scars and is only recommended if a patient desires a less aggressive form of treatment.

Despite the positive results with the IPL and Nd:YAG, there are a limited number of controlled and objective studies in using lasers for hypertrophic and keloid scars. Multicenter, randomized controlled studies that compare laser therapy to other treatment modalities should be established. Additionally, the use of laser and IPL with adjuvant treatments, including intralesional corticosteroids, hydroquinones, 5-fluorouracil, and botulinum toxin should be studied in more detail. More studies into the histology and basic science of hypertrophic scars and the effects of laser therapy and intense pulsed light will hopefully allow us to use the laser at the appropriate time in the wound-healing process to ideally prevent hypertrophic scars and keloids.

References

1. Kontoes PP, Marayiannis KV, Vlachos SP. The use of intense pulsed light in the treatment of scars. Eur J Plast Surg. 2003;25:374–7.
2. Piccolo D, Di Marcantonio D, Crisman G, Cannarozzo G, Sannino M, Chiricozzi A, et al. Unconventional use of intense pulsed light. Biomed Res Int. 2014;2014:618206.
3. Erol OO, Gurlek A, Agaoglu G, Topcuoglu E, Oz H. Treatment of hypertrophic scars and keloids using intense pulsed light (IPL). Aesthet Plast Surg. 2008;32(6):902–9.
4. Han YJJY, Whang KK. Treatment of hypertrophic scars and keloids using intense pulsed light. Korean J Dermatol. 2009;47(4):395–402.

5. Hultman CS, Friedstat JS, Edkins RE. Efficacy of intense pulsed light for the treatment of burn scar dyschromias: a pilot study to assess patient satisfaction, safety, and willingness to pay. Ann Plast Surg. 2015;74(Suppl 4):S204–8.
6. Kim DY, Park HS, Yoon HS, Cho S. Efficacy of IPL device combined with intralesional corticosteroid injection for the treatment of keloids and hypertrophic scars with regards to the recovery of skin barrier function: a pilot study. J Dermatolog Treat. 2015;26(5):481–4.
7. Akaishi S, Koike S, Dohi T, Kobe K, Hyakusoku H, Ogawa R. Nd:YAG laser treatment of keloids and hypertrophic scars. Eplasty. 2012;12:e1.
8. Koike S, Akaishi S, Nagashima Y, Dohi T, Hyakusoku H, Ogawa R. Nd:YAG laser treatment for keloids and hypertrophic scars: an analysis of 102 cases. Plast Reconstr Surg Glob Open. 2014;2(12):e272.
9. Annabathula A, Sekar CS, Srinivas CR. Fractional carbon dioxide, long pulse Nd:YAG and pulsed dye laser in the management of keloids. J Cutan Aesthet Surg. 2017;10(2):76–80.
10. Kumar K, Kapoor BS, Rai P, Shukla HS. In-situ irradiation of keloid scars with Nd:YAG laser. J Wound Care. 2000;9(5):213–5.
11. Sherman R, Rosenfeld H. Experience with the Nd:YAG laser in the treatment of keloid scars. Ann Plast Surg. 1988;21(3):231–5.
12. Abergel RP, Dwyer RM, Meeker CA, Lask G, Kelly AP, Uitto J. Laser treatment of keloids: a clinical trial and an in vitro study with Nd:YAG laser. Lasers Surg Med. 1984;4(3):291–5.
13. Al-Mohamady Ael S, Ibrahim SM, Muhammad MM. Pulsed dye laser versus long-pulsed Nd:YAG laser in the treatment of hypertrophic scars and keloid: a comparative randomized split-scar trial. J Cosmet Laser Ther. 2016;18(4):208–12.
14. Rossi A, Lu R, Frey MK, Kubota T, Smith LA, Perez M. The use of the 300 microsecond 1064 nm Nd:YAG laser in the treatment of keloids. J Drugs Dermatol. 2013;12(11):1256–62.
15. Chen XE, Liu J, Bin Jameel AA, Valeska M, Zhang JA, Xu Y, et al. Combined effects of long-pulsed neodymium-yttrium-aluminum-garnet laser, diprospan and 5-fluorouracil in the treatment of keloid scars. Exp Ther Med. 2017;13(6):3607–12.
16. Lin L, Guo P, Wang X, Huo R, Li Q, Yin S, et al. Effective treatment for hypertrophic scar with dual-wave-length PDL and Nd:YAG in Chinese patients. J Cosmet Laser Ther. 2019;21:228–33.
17. Bowes LE, Nouri K, Berman B, Jimenez G, Pardo R, Rodriguez L, et al. Treatment of pigmented hypertrophic scars with the 585 nm pulsed dye laser and the 532 nm frequency-doubled Nd:YAG laser in the Q-switched and variable pulse modes: a comparative study. Dermatol Surg. 2002;28(8):714–9.
18. Alam M, Voravutinon N, Warycha M, Whiting D, Nodzenski M, Yoo S, et al. Comparative effectiveness of nonpurpuragenic 595-nm pulsed dye laser and microsecond 1064-nm neodymium:yttrium-aluminum-garnet laser for treatment of diffuse facial erythema: a double-blind randomized controlled trial. J Am Acad Dermatol. 2013;69(3):438–43.
19. Hultman CS, Edkins RE, Wu C, Calvert CT, Cairns BA. Prospective, before-after cohort study to assess the efficacy of laser therapy on hypertrophic burn scars. Ann Plast Surg. 2013;70(5):521–6.
20. Morris V, Murphy LM, Rosenberg M, Rosenberg L, Holzer CE III, Meyer WJ III. Itch assessment scale for the pediatric burn survivor. J Burn Care Res. 2012;33(3):419–24.
21. Goldberg DJ. Current trends in intense pulsed light. J Clin Aesthet Dermatol. 2012;5(6):45–53.
22. Alster TS, Tanzi EL. Hypertrophic scars and keloids: etiology and management. Am J Clin Dermatol. 2003;4(4):235–43.

Laser Management of Acne Scars

Paolo Bonan, Nicola Bruscino, Andrea Bassi, Michela Troiano, Emiliano Schincaglia, and Anne Le Pillouer-Prost

1 Introduction

Acne is a common disorder, the psychological impact of which can be devastating and may result in permanently disfiguring scars. It is characterized by inflammation of the pilosebaceous unit with a great variety of clinical signs divided into inflammatory and non-inflammatory lesions. The pleomorphic variety of signs consists of comedones, papules, pustules, and nodules which primarily appear on the face, back, chest, and shoulders. Inflammatory lesions vary from small papules and pustules to large nodules, while the comedones are non-inflammatory. Although it is often an early manifestation of puberty and its course may be self-limiting, the sequelae can last a lifetime, also with different scar formation. Scarring can be a complication of both non-inflammatory and inflammatory acne. Acneiform scars are the outcomes of compromised collagen production during the natural wound-healing process. The intensity and duration of the inflammation are therefore "good" predictors of the risk of scarring. Although not yet clearly clarified, complex individual modulator factors, which also play a key role, include: metalloproteinases (MMPs) hyperactivity (for atrophic scars), MMPs inhibitor hyperactivity or defect activity (for hypertrophic scars), TGF-β subunits abnormalities, interleukins (IL) abnormalities, notably IL-6, and keratinocytes abnormalities that influence the regulation of fibroblast activity. Abnormalities of numerous cell-to-cell or cell-to-cytokine interactions are also involved in tissue inflammation and wound healing. A genetic family susceptibility is possible but the exact mode of transmission is unknown. Post-acne scarring is more frequent in phototype V and VI. It is also more frequent if the acne is excoriated [1, 2].

P. Bonan · N. Bruscino (✉) · A. Bassi · M. Troiano · E. Schincaglia
Laser Cutaneous Cosmetic and Plastic Surgery Unit, Villa Donatello Clinic, Florence, Italy
e-mail: pbonan@vodafone.it

A. Le Pillouer-Prost
Service de Dermatologie, Hôpital Privé Clairval, Marseille, France

2 Review of the Evidence

Acne scars can be divided into three different types: atrophic, hypertrophic depending on the loss or gain of collagen, and red-pigmented macular acne scars (strictly speaking these are not "scars" due to being transient).

Atrophic acne scars are related to particular inflammatory mediators and enzymatic degradation of collagen fibers and fat. Atrophic acne scars are the most common (80–90% of all acne scars patients), and they can be further divided into the following types: ice-pick scars, rolling scars, boxcar scars, perifollicular elastolysis, and complex scars.

- *Ice-pick scars* or V-shaped scars are deep and extend vertically into the deep dermis or subcutaneous tissue, with an opening always wider than the deeper infundibulum. So, they appear as deep, vertical epithelialized punctiform holes (2 mm). They are too deep to be reached with conventional skin resurfacing techniques, and complete recovery is usually impossible without the use of treatments entailing dermal remodeling at least 1 mm below the skin surface.
- *Rolling* or M-shaped scars have a rolling appearance on the overlying skin. They are superficial, with an irregular surface, and a diameter > 4 mm. Although they tend to be shallow, the subdermal tether precludes treatment from the upper surface. Correction of the subdermal component is essential for successful treatment.
- *Boxcar scars* or U-shaped scars are round or oval depressions with sharply demarcated vertical edges and a diameter of 2–4 mm. They are clinically wider at the surface than ice-pick scars and may be shallow (0.1–0.5 mm) or deep (>0.5 mm).
- *Perifollicular elastolysis*: small, round, white thoracic spots with a follicle in the center with a soft texture, probably due to the presence of elastase secreting epidermidis staphylococci.
- *Complex scars*: associating cords, bridges, intra-dermal epithelialized tunnels, multipore comedones, and often a persistent inflammatory disease.

K. Shokrollahi (ed.), *Laser Management of Scars*, https://doi.org/10.1007/978-3-030-52919-2_10

Hypertrophic scars are divided into two types:

- *Simple*: not exceeding the margins of the initial lesions, usually regressive after 12–18 months.
- *Keloid*: exceeding the margins, more frequent in the prethoracical region, the back, or the mandible.

Sometimes the different types of scars can be observed in the same patients and it can be very difficult to differentiate between them [3].

In a more educational way a scale of scores, called ECCA, was published by Pr Dreno and colleagues in 2007, established in accordance with the active disease scale (ECLA) [4]. This is a very useful scale for clinical studies and clinical practice with four groups for atrophic PAS (ice-pick scars, superficial or deep boxcar scars, superficial or deep rolling scars, perifollicular elastolysis) (Table 1). Several English authors propose other classifications for practical and therapeutic purposes, notably Goodman and colleagues [5, 6], as they take the social impact into account and use a stretching test to estimate the presence or otherwise of underlying fibrous adhesions (Table 2).

Table 1 French ECCA grading scale

Type	Level factor (*a*)	Semi quantitative score (*b*)	Grade (*a* × *b*)
"V-shaped" atrophic scars <2 mm and punctiform (ice-pick scars)	15	0 = no scar 1 = a few scars 2 = limited number 3 = many scars	
"U-shaped" atrophic scars, 2–4 mm, sheer edges (boxcar scars)	20	0 = no scar 1 = a few scars 2 = limited number 3 = many scars	
"M-shaped" atrophic scars, more than 4 mm, superficial, irregular surface (rolling scars)	25	0 = no scar 1 = a few scars 2 = limited number 3 = many scars	
Perifollicular elastolysis	30	0 = absent 1 = mild 2 = moderate 3 = intense	
Subgrading 1			
Hypertrophic and inflammatory <2 years of age	40	0 = no scar 1 = a few scars 2 = limited number 3 = many scars	
Keloïds/hypertrophic >2 years of age	50	0 = no scar 1 = a few scars 2 = limited number 3 = many scars	
Subgrading 2			
Global score (1 + 2)			

Table 2 English (Goodman) post-acne scarring quantitative grading scale

Type	1–10 lesions	11–20 lesions	>20 lesions
Mild atrophy			
Macular (erythematous or pigmented) Mildly atrophic "dish-like"	1 point	2 points	3 points
Moderate atrophy			
Moderately atrophic "dish-like" Punched out with shallow, small scars <5 mm Shallow but broad atrophic areas	2 points	4 points	6 points
Severe atrophy			
Punched out, deep, normal bases, (<5 mm) Punched out, deep, abnormal bases, (<5 mm) Linear or troughed dermal scar Large and deep	3 points	6 points	9 points
Hypertrophy			
Papular scars	2 points $S^2 < 5$ cm²	4 points S^2: 5–20 cm²	6 points $S^2 > 20$ cm²
Hypertrophy			
Keloids and hypertrophic scars	6 points	12 points	18 points

3 Treatment Methodology

3.1 Non-laser–Based Treatments

The increasing popularity of the use of oral isotretinoin for early treatment of potentially serious forms of acne has led to a reduction in the post-inflammatory outcomes. However, today as in the past, the treatment of post-acneic scars is a difficult challenge for the dermatologist. The main aim is to establish treatment protocols according to the post-acne scars types, scores or ranks. It is essential to be aware of all the therapeutic armamentarium and know how to use specific, combined, and step-by-step treatments. Most of the therapeutic failures, notably for severe atrophic scars, are due to an inadequate evaluation of the lesion's importance [7].

- Intralesional corticosteroid injections are indicated in the treatment of hypertrophic acne scars, especially in the early erythematous phase, thanks to their ability to reduce fibroblast proliferation and promote collagen degradation. Treatment with steroids is generally effective, with improvement reported in 75% of patients and complete flattening in 40%. Development of hypo-pigmentation, dermal atrophy, and telangiectasia is potential sequelae of this type of treatment.
- Treatment with contact cryotherapy has been studied for this type of acne scars. The exact action mechanism is unclear; however, it is assumed that the physical damage caused by freezing and thrombosis leads to collagen restructuring. According to literature, it is possible to achieve good or excellent results with cryotherapy in 76% of cases. Permanent pigmentary alterations are possible adverse effects of this type of therapy.
- The "punch excision/elevation" techniques are less often practiced nowadays, and the presence of suture devices means they are not appreciated by patients. They are also contraindicated due to the frequent appearance of skin adherence. Despite this, punch techniques are reported to be efficacious, especially for the treatment of single elements and ice-pick scars.
- Subcision is a useful technique for treating superficial atrophic acne scars. A small needle is inserted into the deep dermis of the healthy skin near the scars and moved back and forth in a fan-like motion under the scar, where it releases fibrous bands at a dermal or deep dermal subcutaneous level. A success rate of 50–60% has been reported in the treatment of rolling scars, and prospective, randomized trials have indicated that short-term subcision outcomes are superior to dermal fillers.
- Traditionally used to enhance and smooth skin texture, chemical peeling has also become widespread over the last two decades. Among all different chemical peelings, preparations, and dilutions, only TCA (trichloroacetic acid) at concentrations of 30 and 70% gives satisfactory results. Pigmentary alterations and additional scar formation are possible side effects. Based on the operator's personal experience, the so-called CROSS technique (high concentration of TCA application on single and selected elements) can minimize the risk of side effects.
- Meso-needling therapy is a new option for the treatment of atrophic acne scars. More recent needling systems (the roller is a drum-shaped device with very fine protruding stainless steel needles) also allow for combining the mechanical action with the application of a topical bio-revitalizing agent such as vitamin C or PRP (platelet-rich plasma), with effective dermal stimulation through the percutaneous collagen induction mechanism. In particular, collagen III is the main type of collagen formed in the early wound-healing phase. It is gradually replaced by collagen I over a period of a year or more resulting in an ongoing tissue remodeling for months after the injury. Skin needling and meso-needling are simple, inexpensive treatment methods for managing post-acne atrophic scars. With this technique, the epidermis remains intact with a reduction in most of the adverse risks. Several studies suggest that it may take months to obtain complete results, as the deposition of new collagen takes place gradually, implying that continued skin microneedling is required to achieve the desired clinical and histological improvement with minimal downtime, side effects, and complications.
- A low-viscosity non-animal stabilized hyaluronic acid (NASHA) dermal filler, 20 mg/mL hyaluronic acid (HA) gel, injected in micro-doses into the dermis, may be a useful new approach for improving the appearance of depressed facial acne scars, as well as rolling scars and boxcar scars. Immediate visual improvement is usually observed in all the lesions, while the side effects are usually limited to transient pinpoint bleeding at the injection sites.

All these treatments can provide a valuable support to physical treatments which stimulate the dermis not only through mechanical damage but also through heat damage as with the radiofrequency technique that creates an electric current in the dermis.

3.2 Laser-Based Treatments

Numerous invasive approaches have been suggested for the treatment of each scar types.

Various lasers or lamps can be used for post-acne scars care:

- Ablative lasers: CO_2, Erbium 2940 nm, Erbium 2790 nm (traditional or fractional mode).
- Non-ablative lasers: vascular or pigmentary lasers or intense pulsed lights, infrared lasers (traditional or fractional mode) [8, 9].

3.3 Ablative Lasers

Skin resurfacing using ablative lasers such as 10,600 nm CO_2 and 2940 nm Er:YAG laser have shown the greatest clinical improvements for acne scars; nevertheless, due to the complete vaporization of the epidermis and the variable thermal damage to the dermis, prolonged healing time, and significant associated risks are often reported. Ablative resurfacing with *CO_2 laser* has always been considered the gold standard for treating wrinkles, skin damage from photoaging, and post-acne scars, with up-to-date scanners and various numbers of passes per session. Results were usually very good or excellent but frightening adverse effects were also reported [10–12]. This laser is, the first and by far, the most effective laser for severe atrophic PAS. It replaced mechanical dermabrasion and chemical peeling, but its prolonged healing phase and morbidity haunted numerous patients and practitioners. The greatest fear with this laser is the incidence of permanent hypopigmentation, scarrings, and bacterial and viral infections. CO_2 lasers were preferred for more severe atrophy or mature subjects with skin laxity, while Erbium lasers were added to the armamentarium when a purely ablative effect was desired. *Erbium-YAG lasers* were used for mild-to-moderate scars, without fibrous underlying adhesions and for younger subjects [13]. These treatments were carried out under anesthesia: general, regional with sensory nerve blocks or topical with creams, depending on the gravity and extent of the lesions, after an accurate and in-depth discussion with the patient.

The excellent results obtained with this technique have therefore stimulated the research into methods and technologies capable of achieving similar results while reducing downtimes and side effects. Based on these requirements, "fractional laser" resurfacing has been developed [14]. The principle is to create a dense network of microscopic thermal wounds in "tiny wells" in the dermis. These MTZs (micro-thermal zones) and MAZs (micro-ablative zones) are capable of inducing, in and around them, columns of remodeling effect. The depth and width of the columns depend on the wavelength and parameters used. By preserving surrounded tissues and epidermal islands, postoperative after-effects are minimized, reepithelialization is quick and extra facial areas (neck, hands, chest) can be treated.

The *fractional CO_2 laser* (SmartXide[2] DOT/RF, DEKA M.E.L.A., Calenzano, Italy) is equipped with a new scanning system (HiScan DOT/RF) which makes it possible to obtain vertical micro-columns of damage, micro-ablative, and micro-thermal zones (MAZs and MTZs), surrounded by areas of healthy tissue. Depending on the pulse used, the controlled release of heat in the treated micro-areas has an immediate tissue-shrinking effect and generates the stimulation of growth factors, wound repair, and the reorganization of new collagen. Another feature which increases the versatility of this application is the possibility of selecting the distance (DOT spacing) between surrounding MAZs and MTZs, providing a resurfacing effect similar to the ablative technique with reduced spacing, or the more typical fractional effect, with greater spacing between DOTs. The versatility of this device also derives from the "Smart Pulse mode," a function that allows physicians to obtain two different effects in the target area to be treated, depending on the patient's needs and the type of treatment required, namely, "the ablative effect" and the "thermal effect." The first, which depends mainly on the power (Watts), is achieved with a fast release of high energy to the tissue causing rapid ablation of the epidermis and more superficial dermal layers. Instead, the "thermal effect" depends mainly on the dwell time (μs) during which the heating of the deeper layers of the skin spreads to the surrounding areas and deeper areas of the micro-thermal zone (MTZ), continuing the laser effect. Another important function that we use is the novel "Pulse Stacking mode." Each treatment session consists of numerous successive and consecutive pulses [1–5] in the same point without moving the scanner ("scalpel effect"). This function allows deeper penetration, thanks to the possibility of repeating the laser emissions with the same parameters on one DOT before moving on to the next DOT during the same scanner passage. With the fractional CO_2 treatment, the epidermis receives a sort of micro-ablation and heals in 24–48 h: the epidermal tissue recovery occurs rapidly via keratinocyte migration and extrusion of the damaged cells to the borders of the ablative and thermal zones; the keratinocyte migration occurs, thanks to the presence of "a reservoir" of partially differentiated cells with a high turnover and high mitotic index that are able to repair the tissue deprivation; the epidermal stratus corneum acts as a natural bandage that protects the tissue from noxious external factors while the treatment effects continue in the deeper dermis. An acute phase occurs in the dermis with the releasing of numerous proinflammatory cytokines and mediators, with only moderate collagen fiber shrinkage and oedema. The damaged dermal tissue is massed in columns of debris which move through the epidermis to the stratus corneum and then exfoliate. After this first phase, there is a proliferative phase with the recruitment of fibroblasts and deposition of new type III collagen fibers and dermal matrix; the last phase is characterized by collagen remodeling, when the thinner type III collagen fibers are replaced by type I collagen fibers [15–19]. The new laser systems (SmartXide[2] DOT/RF) simultaneously deliver laser and bipolar radiofrequency (Fig. 1); the latter is able to amplify and enhance the effects of the CO_2 laser by remodeling the tissue in-depth, toning flabbiness, and stimulating fibroblast activity to produce new collagen. Previous histological studies have in fact confirmed the presence of thickened, shortened collagen fibrils after bipolar radiofrequency treatments and an increased collagen I upregulation has been observed through the northern blot analysis. It has therefore been demonstrated how fractional CO_2 laser and radiofrequency are able to induce similar histological modifications in the superficial layers of the skin. The simultaneous emission of CO_2 fractional laser and radiofrequency currents yields several significant beneficial effects. In particular, there is a transfer of energy from the surface to the deeper layers with a more uniform lateral diffusion of the bio-stimulation. The laser–radiofrequency combination minimizes the amount of energy required from each system to achieve the desired results, decreasing the possibilities of side effects. The recovery times are between 3 and 5 days in nearly all patients, and the erythema usually never lasts longer than 5 days, showing a reduction in superficial hyperaemia. The average downtime for the fractional CO_2 laser/bipolar radiofrequency device is 4–5 days, which is a slight reduction compared to previous results using fractional CO_2 laser alone. Faster healing allows patients to return to a normal life in public within the first week after the laser session, since there are no marked side effects to hide or tolerate. Despite a few predictable side effects like erythema and oedema, the majority of patients are usually very satisfied, which suggests that the low downtime and side effects associated with the laser procedure are well tolerated, thanks to the degree of improvement achieved at the end of the treatments (Figs. 2, 3, 4, and 5).

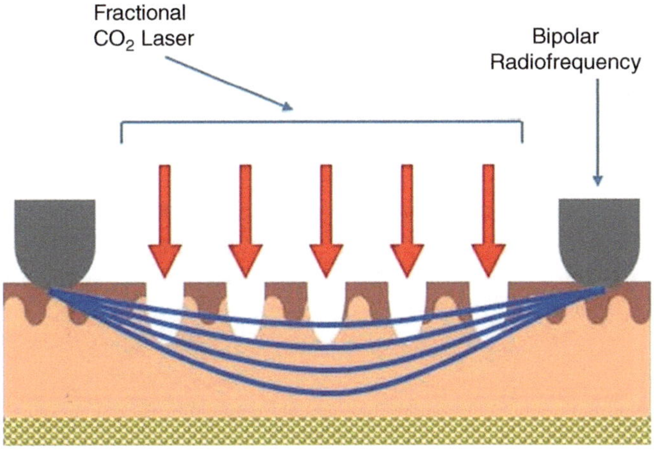

Fig. 1 Synergy between fractional CO_2 laser and bipolar radiofrequency current

The mechanism, through which ablative fractional lasers combined with bipolar radiofrequency are able to improve the appearance of acne scars, is still in part understood. We have conducted previous detailed studies on the cytokine pathway of tissue repair after fractional CO_2 laser session, monitoring the cytokines release at different times (Table 3). In these studies, we noted that a multitude of growth factors and cytokines are present at the wound site; after skin irradiation the dynamics of these vary over time, and the quality and sequential secretion of these cytokines are extremely important for achieving good quality wound repair. The typical cytokines most frequently expressed after the fractional CO_2 laser play a key role in the scar scenario; the vasculogenesis and microangiogenesis are induced by the fractional CO_2 laser effect on cytokines like VEGF and bFGF; the

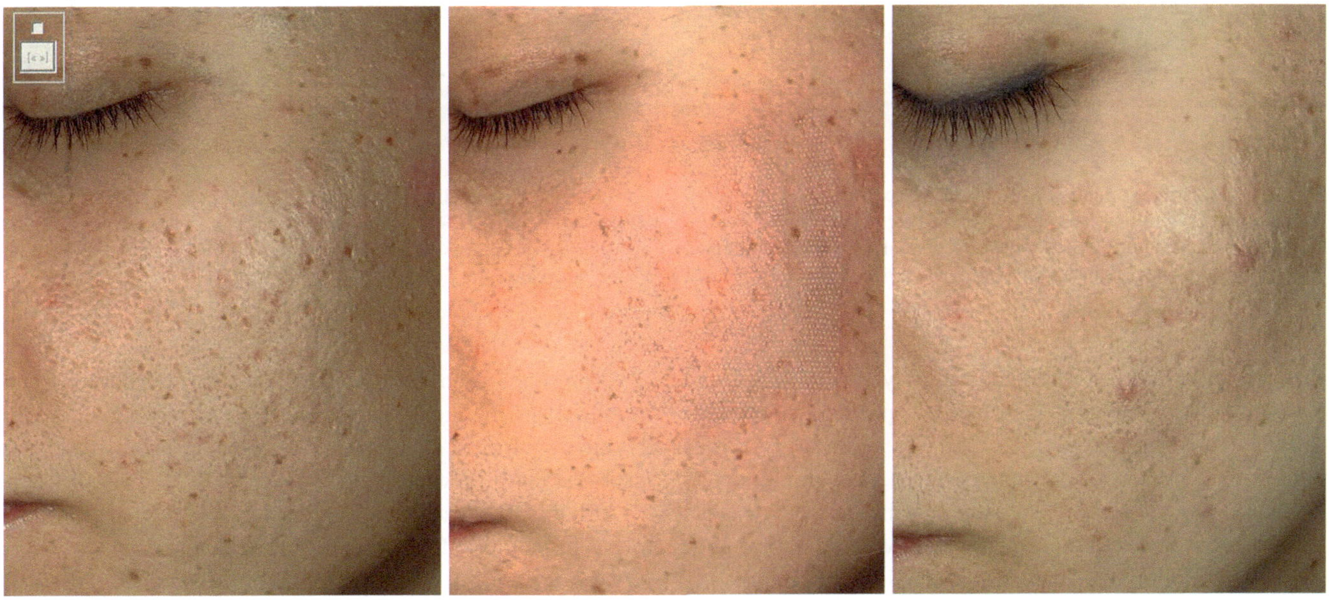

Fig. 2 A 27-year-old girl with ice-pick acne scars previously after numerous sessions of deep peeling with only partial results. The girl was treated with a fractional CO_2 laser combined with radiofrequency (simultaneously delivery of laser and bipolar radiofrequency), SmartXide[2] DOT/RF, with the following parameters: Power 10 W, Dwell Time (DT) 800 μs, Dot Spacing 700 μm, Stack 3, RF Power 30 W, and RF Dwell Time 3 s. During the laser session, the maximum overlap was 5–10%. We performed three laser sessions with a time interval of 2 months

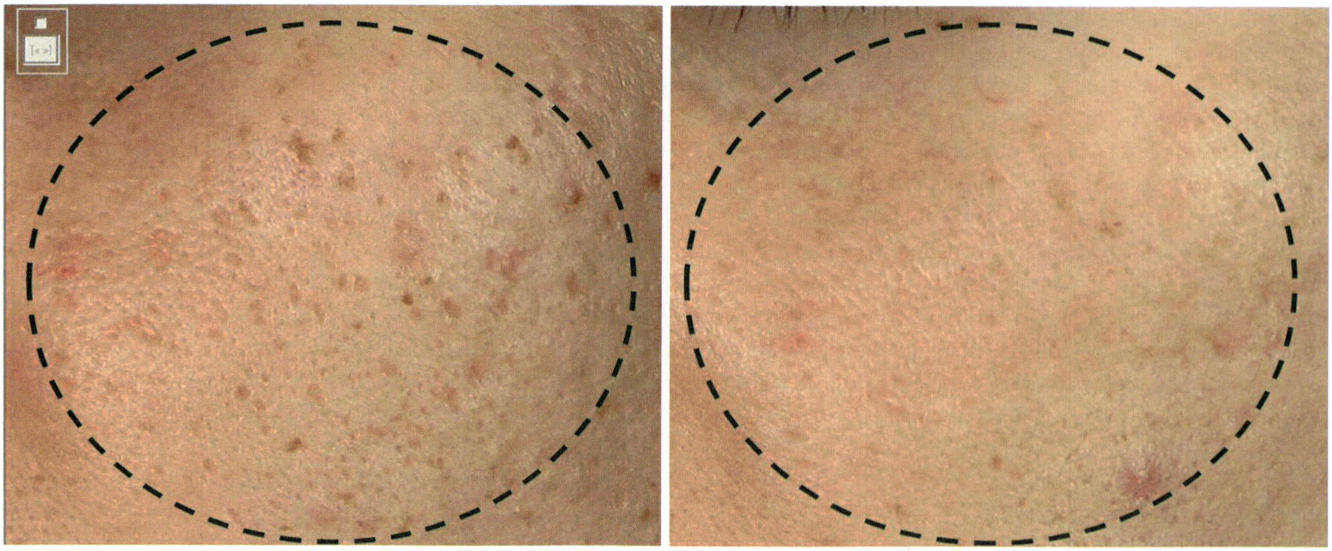

Fig. 3 Detail of the results obtained after three session of SmartXide^2 DOT/RF

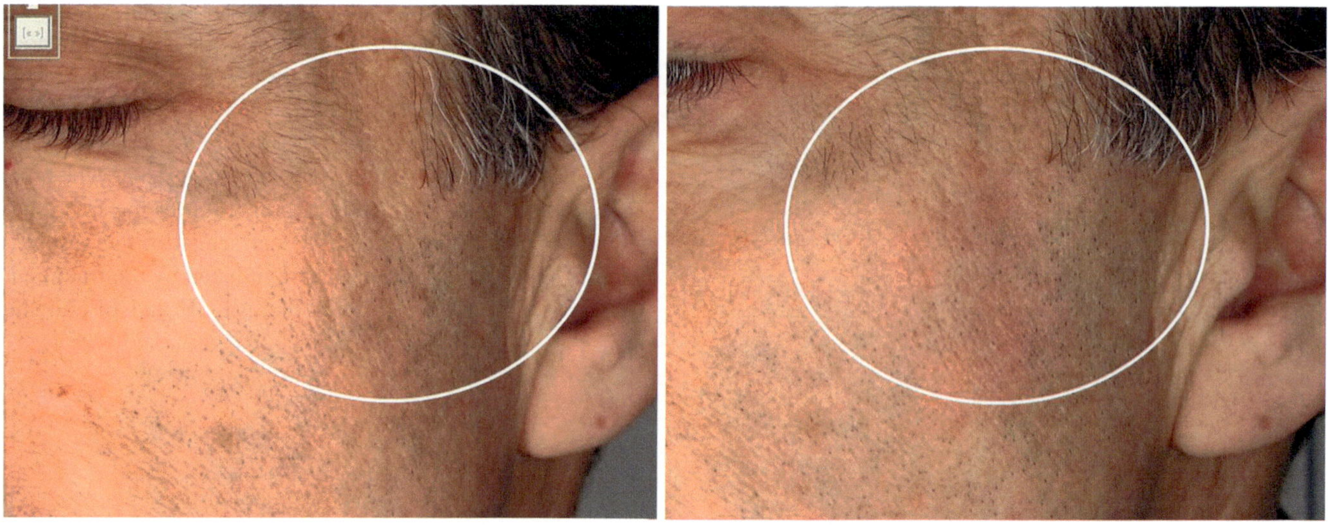

Fig. 4 A 48-year-old male with rolled acne scars previously treated with superficial peelings and intense pulsed light with unsatisfactory results. We treated the patient with a fractional CO_2 laser combined with radiofrequency, SmartXide^2 DOT/RF, with these parameters: Power 10 W, Dwell Time (DT) 800 μs, Dot Spacing 700 μm, Stack 2, RF Power 30 W, and RF Dwell Time 3 s. During the laser session, the maximum overlap was 5–10%. We performed three laser sessions with a time interval of 45–50 days

PDGF release implies a mitogenic activity for fibroblasts and smooth cells, stimulating these cells to produce new extracellular matrix. Moreover, the majority of these cytokines induce the chemotaxis of macrophages and granulocytes, releasing growth factors and other proinflammatory cytokines such as Interleukin-1, Interleukin-6, and Tumor necrosis factor-α, following a cascade mechanism [20, 21].

In this manner, fractional CO_2 laser treatment is able to promote cell replication, and it should potentially be able to balance collagen organization against excessive fibrosis, preventing aberrant wound healing. In vivo human skin histology (presence of dermal spindle cells/myofibroblasts) and immunohistochemical studies (heat shock proteins 72 and 47) have confirmed a persistent collagen remodeling response lasting at least 3 months.

Although the fractional CO_2 laser is an effective and well-tolerated method of treatment for acne scars, patients generally require multiple sessions to achieve significant results, and even then, severe acne scarring is only minimally improved with minimal ablative energies. A specific treatment plan is proposed for each patient depending on PAS severity, phototype, downtime, and budget.

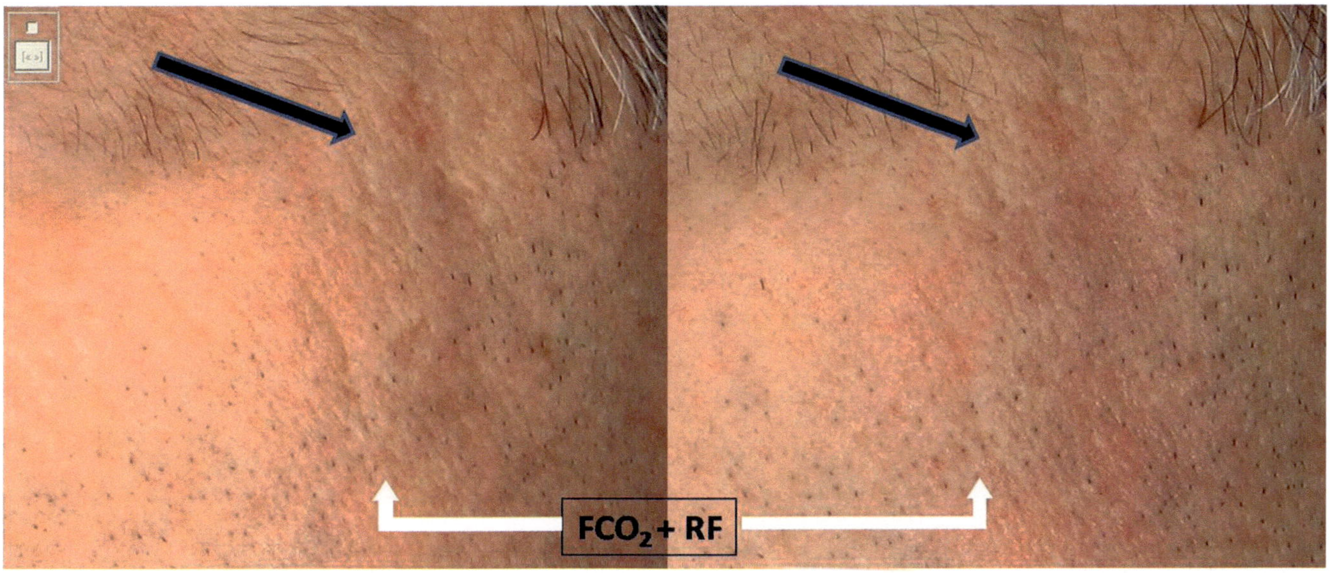

Fig. 5 Detail of the results obtained after three session of SmartXide[2] DOT/RF

Table 3 Cytokine pathway of tissue repair after fractional CO_2 laser session

Cytokines	Functions
TGF-β	• Stimulates matrix proteins (collagen), inhibits protease production, and enhances mitogenesis • Activates the chemotaxis of macrophages and granulocytes and releases proinflammatory cytokines: Interleukin-1, Interleukin-6, and tumor necrosis factor-α
bFGF	• Angiogenetic and mitogenetic activity • Provides the initial stimulation of endothelial cell migration and proliferation • Inhibits collagen production and promotes organized collagen bundles
EGF	• Reepithelization activity (keratinocyte proliferation, keratinocyte marginalization, hyperproliferative wound epidermis)
PDGF	• Chemotactic activity for monocytes, macrophages, and neutrophils • Mitogenic activity for fibroblasts and smooth muscle cells • Stimulates fibroblasts to produce extracellular matrix and to contract collagen matrix
VEGF	• Regulates vasculogenesis and angiogenesis
Vimentin	• Fibroblast protein: Involved in matrix and intercellular substance production

3.4 Non-ablative Lasers

Flashlamp pulsed dye laser (FPDL) (Synchro VasQ, DEKA M.E.L.A., Calenzano, Italy) is a non-ablative laser that has gained an excellent reputation in vascular lesion treatment. It emits a 595-nm wavelength yellow light, near the hemoglobin and oxyhemoglobin absorption peaks, and it is therefore considered the most specific laser currently available for treating superficial vascular lesions. Current indications of this technology have further been extended to include nonvascular lesions but with vascular structural involvement like scars and keloids (Fig. 6). Its combination with fractional CO_2 laser can be very effective, since the latter modulates the release of cytokines normally involved in wound-healing processes, thereby promoting cell replication and the balance of collagen organization against excessive fibrosis, while PDL may limit the perfusion and nutrition of the scar, and consequently its growth. The usual action mechanism of PDL is therefore based on selective thrombosis of vessels with the consequent obliteration of the nutrient supply to the lesions. Due to its effect on the microvessels and consequently on platelet activation, several growth factors are released such as PDGF, TGF-beta, which are powerful fibroblast stimulators. Moreover the hypoperfusion and hypoxia provoked by PDL may also result in neocollagenesis, collagen fibers heating with dissociation of disulfide bonds and subsequent collagen fibers realignment, and the release of histamine or other factors that influence the fibroblast activity [22]. Kuo et al. have also demonstrated that a 585-nm flashlamp pumped pulsed dye laser can modulate the fibroblasts proliferation and type III collagen deposition through the induction of apoptosis, the upregulation of extracellular signal-regulated kinase, and the p38 mitogen-activated protein kinase activity [23].

Moreover, PDL may prove useful for shading off the persistent red macules and the erythematous component of post-

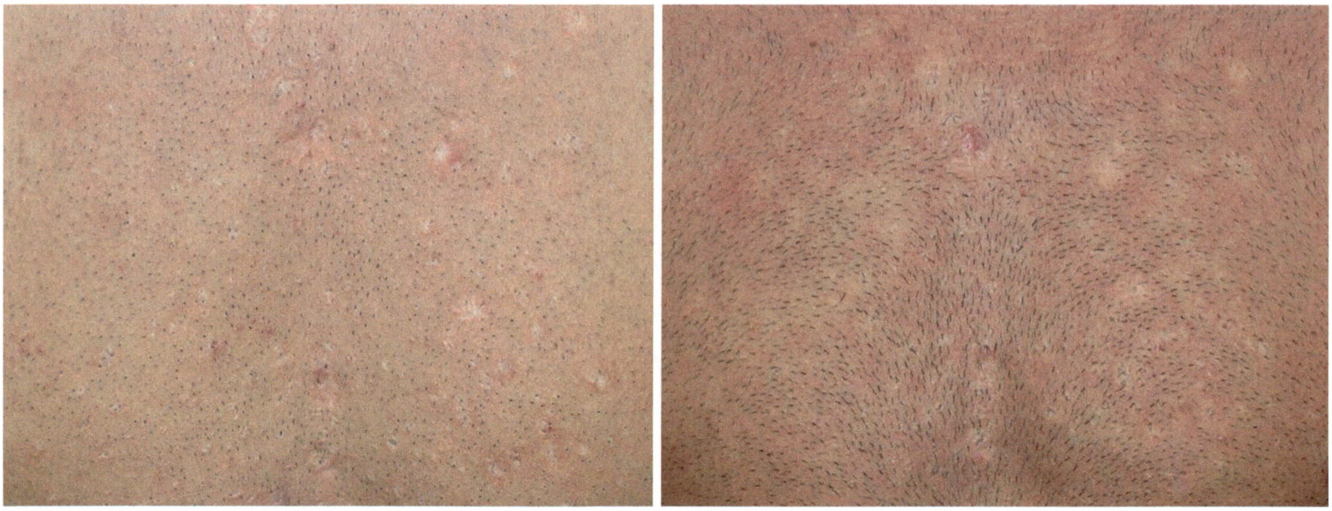

Fig. 6 A 30-year-old man with extensive hypertrophic acne scars on the trunk and chest previously treated for a long period with topical retinoids. The patient was only treated with FPDL (Synchro VasQ) using the following parameters: Fluence 6.5 J/cm^2, Pulse 0.5 ms, and Spot size 10 mm. We performed three laser sessions with a time interval of 45 days

acne scars. The clinical treatment protocol usually consists of 2–4 sessions at 4-week intervals. Relevant side effects such as blisters, crusts, atrophy, scars, are absent in all conditions; many patients show typical PDL-induced side effects like swelling and purpura, which disappear in a few days. The combination of a minimally ablative device like the fractional CO_2 laser with the pulsed dye laser (PDL) may sometimes be suggested, as this achieves promising results without side effects and with a rapid wound healing.

Q-switched Nd:YAG lasers: 1064 nm can be used to treat macules or pigmented scars. Superficial abrasions may be obtained by increasing the sessions for moderate atrophic scars [24].

Numerous *IPL (intense pulsed light)* devices are used for their vascular, pigmentary, or remodeling effects, although literature is inadequate and ambiguous regarding remodeling, and there are currently no scientific proofs of their efficiency. With parameters similar to those used with vascular lasers, they can also be proposed in combined therapies to treat excessive scarring.

Infrared lasers were used in 1998–2000, as their infrared emission leads to a deep light penetration with the possibility of heating the dermis without altering the epidermis. The temperature elevation induces a low-grade inflammatory response and consequently triggers all the cascades of cellular and bio molecular events that can give rise to fibroplasia. However, their often rather modest results are not reproducible from patient to patient [25, 26]. The efficiency may fluctuate, in fact the fibroblastic response seems strongly bound to the patient's genetics, age, degree of solar elastosis, and hormonal and nutritional status. Younger subjects often react better to these techniques. 1064-nm *Nd:YAG lasers* already used for hair removal, leg veins, and other vascular indications seem to give effective results that are at least comparable, or even superior, than those of infrared lasers for scar remodeling [27]. Collagen denaturation and dermis remodeling have been reported. A recent report confirmed this idea with an improvement in the appearance of acne scars, particularly superficial scars, after 1064-nm Nd:YAG sessions, comparable to the 585–595-nm PDL, with significant collagen production and deposition. The authors observed that ice-pick scars and boxcar scars tended to respond better to PDL and Nd:YAG, respectively [22].

Long-term data regarding *non-ablative fractional lasers* for treating acne scars demonstrate promising results (50–75% of improvement in 90% of patients), especially for moderate atrophic PAS [28–32]. Side effects are usually mild and transient: erythema, oedema, dryness, and suntanning appearance. The skin cooling system increases patient comfort and also decreases MTZ size and may interfere with treatment efficiency as has been recently demonstrated by Laubach and colleagues [33]. Histological and immunochemical studies were conducted and reported by two teams in 2006 [34–37]. At the epidermis level, keratinocytes were replaced in 24 h and normal skin restored in 7 days. At the dermis level, the production of collagen III, a strong expression of HSP 70 (first by keratinocytes, and later around the dermis MTZs), and a myofibroblastic response were observed. The main problems with these fractional lasers are the cost of the device and the consumables needed for each session (usually 4–6 sessions) and for these reasons ablative fractional lasers (fractional CO_2 and fractional Erbium laser) are usually preferred by physicians who require effective, more economical laser systems (Table 4) [38–40].

Table 4 Post-acne scars treatment modalities

Type of scar treatment	Ice-pick PAS	Boxcar PAS: Distensible	Boxcar PAS: Non distensible	Rolling PAS	Excessive PAS: Papular	Excessive PAS: Hypertrophic minor keloid	Excessive PAS: Major keloid
Surgery							
Excision	++		++				++
Punch elevation			++				
Subcision				+			
Laser and EBD							
Conventional laser skin resurfacing (LSR)		++	++*	+++			
Non-ablative FL (NAFL)		+		++	+	+	+
Ablative FL (AFL)	++ (fast)	++ (fast)	++* (fast)	+++ (fast)	++	++	++
Bipolar RF (BRF)		+		+	+		
FMR Non-insulated needles		++		++	++		
Fractional RF Insulated-needles	++	++	++*	+	+		
Infrared laser (Nd:Yag LP, 1450, 1540 nm…)		+		+			
AFL CO2 + RF (same device)	+++	+++	++*	+++	+		
LLLT alone						+	+
LLLT combined	+	+	+	+	+	+	+
Vascular laser or lamps						++	+*
Laser or microneedling-assisted drug delivery							
Steroids						+	+
Fillers, cells…		++	++*	++			
Chemical peels							
TCA	+ (cross)	+	+	+			
Phenol	+*	+++	++*	+++			
Fillers, cells, GF…							
Fillers, cells, GF…			++	++			

+: efficient as a unique modality; +* efficient only in combination; *LSR* laser skin resurfacing, *AFL* ablative fractional laser, *FAST* focal acne scar technique, *NAFL* non-ablative fractional laser, *FAST* focal acne scar technique, *LADD* laser-assisted drug delivery, *IL* intralesional, *RF* radiofrequency, *BRF* bipolar radiofrequency, *PDL* pulsed dye laser, *FMR* fractional microneedling radiofrequency, *TCA* trichloroacetic acid, *CROSS* chemical reconstruction of skin scars, *GF* growth factor

4 Clinical Examples

4.1 Ice-Pick Acne Scars

4.2 Rolling Acne Scars

4.3 Hypertrophic Acne Scars

5 Discussion

The basis for successful treatments of post-acne scarring is greater understanding of its pathogenesis, of the genetic reasons why certain people scar and others do not, the inflammatory mediators, and the immunological factors. The classification and grading of both hypertrophic and atrophic diseases must also be known for ensuring optimum management. If the treatment has historically been limited by the morbidity of most treatments with only partial improvement, the development of new techniques, notably lasers which offer more favorable benefit risk profiles, will help practitioners in the management of this common and stressful disorder.

The concept of skin remodeling using minimal or non-ablative light sources has developed rapidly over the last few years. It is widely accepted that these treatments can be integrated in daily practice to combat the cutaneous aging process, but very few reports exist regarding the possibility of treating acne scars according to the same concept. From a biological point of view, the concept of collagen remodeling, which is the goal of every skin rejuvenation treatment, could also be applied to acne scar depressions. Classical treatments of acne scars often give frustrating results even with more invasive modalities, due to the pain and long downtime. The new laser systems have the advantage of being relatively painless, with no risks of adverse reactions. Various laser sources have been developed that stimulate fibroblasts to produce new collagen and influence the collagen fibers realignment with promising clinical results. Moreover, the associated use of these lasers devices limits the perfusion and nutrition of scar tissues, consequently deprives hair growth. Clinical research must still evaluate the benefits of different methods (Table 5).

Table 5 Our suggestions according to the acne scars types

Subtype of scar treatment choices	Ice-pick		Boxcar			Excessive			
	Few	Numerous	Distensible	Non distensible	Rolling	Papular	Hypertrophic minor keloids	Major keloids	Achromic elastolysis
First choice	Punch excision	AFL (FAST) AFL + RF (FAST) Insulated FMR	LSR conventional AFL (FAST) AFL + RF (FAST) RF devices	Surgery Excision Punch elevation	LSR conventional AFL (FAST) AFL + RF (FAST) RF devices	NAFL	Vascular laser (PDL) and AFL (alternatively)	Surgery (revision)	AFL
Second choice	AFL (FAST) AFL + RF (FAST) Insulated FMR TCA-CROSS	TCA-CROSS	Microneedling Chemical peel	LSR (conv.) AFL (FAST) AFL + RF (FAST) Insulated FMR	Microneedling Chemical peel	AFL			UVB
Combined therapies		Surgery and AFL or NAFL and/ or FMR devices	LADD	Surgery and LADD Fillers Autologous cells, PRP, GF..	Subcision LADD Fillers Autologous cells, PRP, GF…		Always: Compression, steroids IL or LADD	Recurrence prevention:Treat the wound bed as a minor keloid	AFL + UVB or sun exposure

LSR laser skin resurfacing, *AFL* ablative fractional laser, *FAST* focal acne scar technique, *NAFL* non-ablative fractional laser, *FAST* focal acne scar technique, *LADD* laser-assisted drug delivery, *IL* intralesional, *RF* radiofrequency, *BRF* bipolar radiofrequency, *PDL* pulsed dye laser, *FMR* fractional microneedling radiofrequency, *TCA* trichloroacetic acid, *CROSS* chemical reconstruction of skin scars, *GF* growth factor

References

1. Chivot M, Pawin H, Beylot C, et al. Acne scars: epidemiology, physiopathology, clinical features and treatment. Ann Dermatol Venereol. 2006;133:813–24.
2. Holland DB, Jeremy AH, Roberts SG, Seukeran DC, Layton AM, Cunliffe WJ. Inflammation in acne scarring: a comparison of the responses in lesions from patients prone and not prone to scar. Br J Dermatol. 2004;150:72–81.
3. Jacob CI, Dover JS, Kaminer MS. Acne scarring:a classification system and review of treatment options. J Am Acad Dermatol. 2001;45:109–17.
4. Dreno B, Khammari A, Orain N, et al. ECCA grading scale :an original validated acne scar grading scale for clinical practice in dermatology. Dermatology. 2007;214:46–51.
5. Goodman GJ, Baron JA. The management of postacne scarring. Dermatol Surg. 2007;33(10):1175–88.
6. Goodman GJ, Baron JA. Postacne scarring-a qualitative global scarring grading system. Dermatol Surg. 2006;32:1458–66.
7. Levy LL, Zeichner JA. Management of acne scarring, part II: a comparative review of non-laser based, minimally invasive approaches. Am J Clin Dermatol. 2012;13(5):331–40.
8. Sobanko JF, Alster TS. Management of acne scarring part I: a comparative review of laser surgical approach. Am J Clin Dermatol. 2012;13(5):319–30.
9. Alster TS, Zaulyanov L. Laser scar revision: a review. Dermatol Surg. 2007;33:131–40.
10. Nanni CA, Alster TS. Complications of carbon dioxide laser resurfacing. An evaluation of 500 patients. Dermatol Surg. 1998;24:315–20.
11. Garret AB, Dufresne RG Jr, Ratz JL, Berlin AJ. Carbon dioxide laser treatment of pitted acne scarring. J Dermatol Surg Oncol. 1990;16:737–40.
12. Walia S, Alster TS. Prolonged clinical and histologic effects from CO_2 laser resurfacing of atrophic acne scars. Dermatol Surg. 1999;25(12):926–30.
13. Woo SH, Park JH, Kye YC. Resurfacing of different types of facial acne scar with short-pulsed, variable-pulsed, and dual-mode Er:YAG laser. Dermatol Surg. 2004;30(4 Pt 1):488–93.
14. Manstein D, Herron GS, Sink RK, Tanner AH, Anderson RR. Fractional photothermolysis: a new concept for cutaneous remodeling using microscopic patterns of thermal injury. Lasers Surg Med. 2004;34:426–38.
15. Chapas AM, Brightman L, Sukal S, et al. Successful treatment of acneiform scarring with CO_2 ablative fractional resurfacing. Lasers Surg Med. 2008;40(6):381–6.
16. Walgrave SE, Ortiz AE, MacFalls HAT, et al. Evaluation of a novel fractional resurfacing device for treatment of acne scarring. Lasers Surg Med. 2009;41(2):122–7.
17. Gotkin RH, Sarnoff DS, Cannarozzo G, Sadick NS, Alexiades-Armenakas M. Ablative skin resurfacing with a novel microablative CO_2 laser. J Drugs Dermatol. 2009;8(2):138–44.
18. Reinholz M, Schwaiger H, Heppt MV, et al. Comparison of two kinds of lasers in the treatment of acne scars. Facial Plast Surg. 2015;31(5):523–31.
19. Omi T, Numano K. The role of the CO_2 laser and fractional CO_2 laser in dermatology. Laser Ther. 2014;23(1):49–60.
20. Prignano F, Campolmi P, Bonan P, et al. Fractional CO_2 laser: a novel therapeutic device upon photobiomodulation of tissue remodelling and cytokine pathway of tissue repair. Dermatol Ther. 2009;22:s8–s15.
21. Prignano F, Bonciani D, Campolmi P, Cannarozzo G, Bonan P, Lotti T. A study of frcational CO_2 laser resurfacing: the best fluences through a clinical, histological, and ultrastructural evaluation. J Cosmet Dermatol. 2011;10:210–6.
22. Lee DH, Choi YS, Min SU, Yoon MY, Suh DH. Comparison of a 585 nm pulsed dye laser and a 1064 nm Nd-YAG laser for the treatment of acne scars: a randomized split-face clinical study. J Am Acad Dermatol. 2009;60(5):801–7.
23. Kuo YR, Wu WS, Jeng SF, et al. Activation of ERK and p38 kinase mediated keloid fibroblast apoptosis after flashlamp pulsed dye laser treatment. Laser Surg Med. 2005;36:31–7.
24. Friedman PM, Jih MH, Skover GR, Payonk GS, Kimyai-Asadi A, Geronemus RG. Treatment of atrophic facial acne scars with the 1064-nm Q-switched Nd:YAG laser: six-month follow-up study. Arch Dermatol. 2004;140(11):1337–41.
25. Tanzi EL, Alster TS. Comparison of a 1450-nm diode laser and a 1320-nm Nd:YAG laser in the treatment of atrophic facial scars: a prospective clinical and histologic study. Dermatol Surg. 2004;30:152–7.
26. Bhatia AC, Dover JS, Arndt KA, Stewart B, Alam M. Patient satisfaction and reported long-term therapeutic efficacy associated with 1,320 nm Nd:YAG laser treatment of acne scarring and photoaging. Dermatol Surg. 2006;32(3):346–52.
27. Keller R, Belda Júnior W, Valente NY, Rodrigues CJ. Nonablative 1,064-nm Nd:YAG laser for treating atrophic facial acne scars: histologic and clinical analysis. Dermatol Surg. 2007;33(12):1470–6.
28. Alster TS, Tanzi EL, Lazarus M. The use of fractional laser photothermolysis for the treatment of atrophic scars. Dermatol Surg. 2007;33(3):295–9.
29. Hasegawa T, Matsukura T, Mizuno Y, Suga Y, Ogawa H, Ikeda S. Clinical trial of a laser device called fractional photothermolysis system for acne scars. J Dermatol. 2006;33(9):623–7.
30. Lee HS, Lee JH, Ahn GY, et al. Fractional photothermolysis for the treatment of acne scars: a report of 27 Korean patients. J Dermatolog Treat. 2008;19(1):45–9.
31. Chrastil B, Glaich AS, Goldberg LH, Friedman PM. Second generation 1550 nm fractional photothermolysis for the treatment of acne scars. Dermatol Surg. 2008;34(10):1327–32.
32. Cho SB, Lee JH, Choi MJ, Lee KY, Oh SH. Efficacy of the fractional photothermolysis system with dynamic operating mode on acne scars and enlarged facial pores. Dermatol Surg. 2009;35(1):108–14.
33. Laubach H, Chan HH, Rius F, Anderson RR, Mainstein D. Effects of skin temperature on lesion size in fractional photothermolysis. Lasers Surg Med. 2007;39(1):14–8.
34. Laubach HJ, Tannous Z, Anderson RR, Manstein D. Skin responses to fractional photothermolysis. Laser Surg Med. 2006;38:142–9.
35. Hantash BM, Bedi VP, Sudireddy V, Struck SK, Herron GS, Chan KF. Laser-induced transepidermal elimination of dermal content by fractional photothermolysis. J Biomed Opt. 2006;11(4):041115.
36. Hantash BM, Bedi VP, Chan KF, Zachary CB. Ex vivo histological characterization of a novel ablative fractional resurfacing device. Lasers Surg Med. 2007;39(2):87–95.
37. Hantash BM, Bedi VP, Kapadia B, et al. In vivo histological evaluation of a novel ablative fractional resurfacing device. Lasers Surg Med. 2007;39(2):96–107.
38. Bernstein EF. Double-pass, low-fluence laser treatment using a large spot-size 1450 nm laser improves acne. Lasers Surg Med. 2009;41(2):116–21.
39. Degitz K. Nonablative fractional lasers: acne scars and other indications. Hautarzt. 2015;66(10):753–6.
40. Shah S, Alam M. Laser resurfacing pearls. Semin Plast Surg. 2012;26(3):131–6.

Strategies for Keloid and Hypertrophic Scars with Lasers

Gerd G. Gauglitz and Julian Poetschke

1 Introduction

Currently, first-line treatment options for hypertrophic scarring and keloids are mainly dominated by conservative treatment approaches, such as intralesional triamcinolone acetonide injections in combination with cryotherapy or silicone gel sheeting, which have proven reliable over years of clinical use [1]. Novel techniques such as intralesional 5-FU, intralesional cryotherapy, and various lasers have successfully been tested in well-designed trials and already have or may extend the current spectrum of excessive scar treatment in the future. Particularly, the latter do play an increasingly important role in everyday clinical routine. To date, four distinct wavelengths are mainly being employed for both the prevention and treatment of hypertrophic scars and keloids.

2 Examining the Evidence

2.1 Pulsed Dye Laser (PDL)

In 1995, the efficacy of the PDL for the treatment of sternal keloids was first stipulated by Alster et al. who demonstrated clear improvements of scar parameters like scar height, skin surface texture, and erythema, as well as symptoms like pruritus [2]. The mode of action of the pulsed dye laser is based on the selective targeting of oxyhemoglobin. Its absorption of the laser energy leads to coagulation within the blood vessel, and the resulting damage to the microvascular network causes hypoperfusion and hypoxia in the surrounding tissue. The biochemical changes include TGF-β1 suppression, which causes the halt of fibroblast proliferation and the increase of the production of antiproliferative agents such as MMP-13, ERK, and p38 kinase [3, 4]. Currently recommended treatment regimes for the treatment of hypertrophic scars and keloids include the use of non-overlapping laser pulses with fluences ranging from 6.0 to 7.5 J/cm^2 (7 mm spot) or from 4.5 to 5.5 J/cm^2 (10 mm spot) [5]. For the improvement of scar properties like color, height, pliability, and texture, Alster et al. recommend two to six treatment sessions [6]. The results achieved in this study, however, could not be reproduced in several subsequent trials [7]. Indeed, when employing longer follow-up observation, some case-control studies could not find any significant differences between treated and untreated groups [8, 9]. Currently, most studies examining the effect of the PDL suffer from methodological problems such as small case numbers, insufficiently short follow-up periods, uncontrolled study algorithms, and a lack of differentiation between keloids and hypertrophic scarring or further information on the treated scars. Thus, the level of evidence for the efficacy of pulsed dye laser treatment for keloids and hypertrophic scars is relatively low [10]. However, current research and clinical experience on hypertrophic scar and keloid treatment show a distinct efficacy of the PDL, leading to current international guidelines recommending it as a first- or second-line therapy for immature and erythematous hypertrophic scars and linear hypertrophic scars. It has also been approved as a secondary treatment option for erythematous and severely pruritic keloids [1, 11–15]. Side effects are generally mild and include predominantly purpura, usually persisting for 7–14 days. Depending on the energy density employed, vesicles and crusts may occur. Longer persisting hyperpigmentation occurs particularly in darker skin types and is less frequent with the use of the wavelength 595 nm than with 585 nm [1].

Next to treatment of already existing hypertrophic scars and keloids, the pulsed dye laser has also been described as an effective tool to improve the quality and cosmetic appearance of surgical scars in skin types I–IV when starting treatments on the day of suture removal [16]. As demonstrated by the

G. G. Gauglitz (✉)
Department of Dermatology and Allergy, Ludwig-Maximilian-University, Munich, Germany
e-mail: gerd.gauglitz@med.uni-muenchen.de

J. Poetschke
Department of Dermatology and Allergy, Ludwig-Maximilian-University, Munich, Germany

Department of Plastic and Handsurgery, Burn Center, Klinikum St. Georg gGmbH, Leipzig, Germany
e-mail: mail@julian-poetschke.de

K. Shokrollahi (ed.), *Laser Management of Scars*, https://doi.org/10.1007/978-3-030-52919-2_11

same group, both the 585- and 595-nm PDL treatments appear to be effective in improving the appearance and normalizing the vascularity and pliability of postoperative scars [17]. Author recommendations included three laser sessions at 4-week intervals starting on the day of suture removal.

2.2 Nd:YAG

Next to the PDL, the Nd:YAG laser has been highlighted as a potential means to improve hypertrophic scars and keloids. While similar to the PDL when it comes to its mode of action, the Nd:YAG laser possesses improved skin penetration when compared to the PDL. Its efficacy, however, is still reduced in greater depths. Patients being treated with the Nd:YAG laser describe a prickling sensation during treatment and posttreatment side effects include mostly erythema and swelling [18]. The Nd:YAG could demonstrate improvement of scar height, pliability, vascularity, and pigmentation in a small pilot study by Cho et al. [18] Later on, its significant improvement of hypertrophic scarring and keloids could be shown in a larger patient cohort (102 patients) from Japan. While successful though, recurrence rates of up to 52.9% after 6 months were reported [19]. In another study, comparing the combined use of the Nd:YAG laser and intralesional corticosteroids with the sole injection of intralesional corticosteroids, superior results for the laser-assisted treatment plan could be shown [20].

Overall, however, current research has not yet produced enough data to satisfyingly prove the adequacy of the Nd:YAG for hypertrophic scar and keloid treatment. Its use is not yet guideline-recommended, while its adaption in circumstances similar to those for PDL treatment might still prove fruitful.

2.3 Ablative Lasers: Carbon Dioxide (CO_2) Laser and Er:YAG

Ablative lasers like the carbon dioxide (CO_2) laser or the Er:YAG laser allow for very exact and controlled ablation of tissue. The Er:YAG laser features a wavelength of 2940 nm which leads to significant energy absorption into water. Therefore, heat transfer into the surrounding tissue and heat necrosis are uncommon, when using the Er:YAG laser. The CO_2 laser (10,600 nm), on the other hand, relies on the transfer of heat into the surrounding tissue, allowing it to coagulate blood vessels, as it cuts the tissue, thus facilitating more extensive tissue ablation. Side effects like crusting, weeping, and erythema are common with both lasers. Pigmentation disorders, too, can occur, though they are frequently more pronounced with the CO_2 laser.

Recently, the use of ablative lasers in a fractional mode has become more and more popular. It allows the splitting of the laser beam into a grid of smaller beams, thus leaving intact skin islets. Fractional photothermolysis is based upon the scientific concept of creating microscopic thermal wounds deep to the surface of the skin, which allow for tissue contraction, stimulation of collagen, and rapid wound healing. Since studies could prove a positive effect on collagen remodeling and the equilibrium of heat shock proteins, MMP-1, TGF-β2, and β3 as well as bFGF, the use of fractional lasers for the treatment of postsurgical and hypertrophic (burn) scars has been advocated by experts [21–23]. Randomized clinical trials comparing fractional ablative laser treatment with pulsed dye laser therapy for the postoperative treatment of surgical scars showed superior results for the fractional ablative approach [24, 25]. Ultrapulsed fractional CO_2 laser resurfacing could also be shown to be superior than dermabrasion for the improvement of severe posttraumatic and surgical scars [26]. In the treatment of burn scars, fractional CO_2 laser therapy has proven efficacious in improving structural properties of the scarring as well as their clinical aspect. In comparison with non-ablative devices, fewer treatment sessions are required, thus making fractional ablative laser treatment the preferred method [27–29].

Overall, current guidelines are cautious in regard to purely ablative laser treatment for hypertrophic scars, since systematic clinical research data confirming their suitability and safety is still largely missing. However, fractional ablative laser treatment (mostly CO_2) may be considered as a first- or second-line option to flatten inactive hypertrophic (burn) scarring and to loosen contractures [1, 13–15]. Although not included in current guidelines, recent results highlight the importance of fractional ablative and non-ablative lasers for the prevention of unpleasant scarring. Similarly to the concept of utilizing a PDL early after wounding in order to improve the scar healing process, protocols recommend initiation of these treatments after suture removal employing moderate energies. Even though initial results seem promising, more objective data is needed in order to draw final conclusions from this novel approach.

Currently, ablative laser treatment does not play a large role in keloid treatment. Since keloids are prone to recur, primary ablative treatment is not recommended. When combined with adequate prophylactic measures, it can be considered to debulk larger keloids or as a secondary measure in therapy refractory scars, though [1, 15].

3 Treatment Methodology

Depending on the type of scar and associated symptoms, the choice of the respective laser may vary. While erythematous elevated scars may benefit from PDL or Nd:YAG laser treatments, due to the underlying mode of action the limited penetration depth should be taken into consideration before initiating any therapy. Thus, particularly with inflamed keloids, the initiation of an anti-inflammatory treatment such as intralesional triamcinolone acetonide may be useful before starting laser therapy. Here, next to the anti-inflammatory effect, the main goal is to reduce the scar height, which may be more effectively achieved when combined with cryotherapy (patient 1). Importantly, especially when it comes to treatment of keloids, often multiple treatments are necessary in order to achieve satisfying results.

With older linear or widespread hypertrophic scars, frequently, an improvement of scar texture, pliability, and softening of scar tissue is warranted. Here, fractional lasers do play an increasingly important role. Although both, ablative and non-ablative, devices may be employed, current guidelines are in favor of the fractional CO_2 due to its penetration depth (up to 4 mm) and the ability to ablate excessive scar tissue. As with most modalities, multiple sessions are needed and due to the fact that the collagen remodeling process is initiated, final results are mainly seen months after the last procedure (patient 2).

4 Clinical Examples

Patient 1: A 29-year-old healthy woman with Fitzpatrick Skin Type II presented for treatment of a moderately large keloid over the V-region of her chest, which had developed after the excision of a histiocytoma. The patient reported that cryotherapy every 4 weeks for a total of 3 months had not shown any improvement but rather led to an increase in size and pruritus (Fig. 1a, b). After careful discussion of the possible treatment options, potential side effects, and after signing informed consent, a combined approach of spray cryotherapy directly followed by injection of triamcinolone acetonide (TAC, 10 mg/ml) was initiated and repeated monthly. Within 12 weeks, the protrusion of the keloid gradually decreased (Fig. 1c) and marked improvement of pruritus was noted. To further improve the appearance of the skin lesion, PDL was suggested for the treatment of the residual erythema and some telangiectasia. Treatments with a PDL (Candela Vbeam Perfecta, Candela Corp., Wayland, MA) were started 4 weeks after the last steroid injection at 585 nm wavelength delivering a fluence of 7.0 J/cm^2 with pulse duration of 1500 ms and 7 mm spot size at 4- to 5-week intervals. In order to prevent possible reactivation of the keloid by the laser treatment, the patient administered a silicone gel to the affected area twice daily beginning 1 week after each laser session. After four dye laser applications and continuous administration of the silicone gel, the keloid became flat and erythema faded (Fig. 1d). A follow-up examination 6 months later did not reveal any signs of recurrence or reactivation of the successfully treated keloid (Fig. 1e, f).

Patient 2: A 27-year-old healthy female with Fitzpatrick Skin Type V seeked help for improvement of widespread hypertrophic scars which have been the consequence of a third degree burn more than 5 years ago. She had undertaken numerous reconstructive surgical procedures but was to date mostly worrying about the uneven scar texture, pliability, and tension (Fig. 2a). After careful discussion of the existing options in order to improve scar surface and overall appearance, a fractional CO_2 treatment was initiated. Due to the skin colur, a patch area was treated first with representative settings in order to control for potential risk of hypo- or

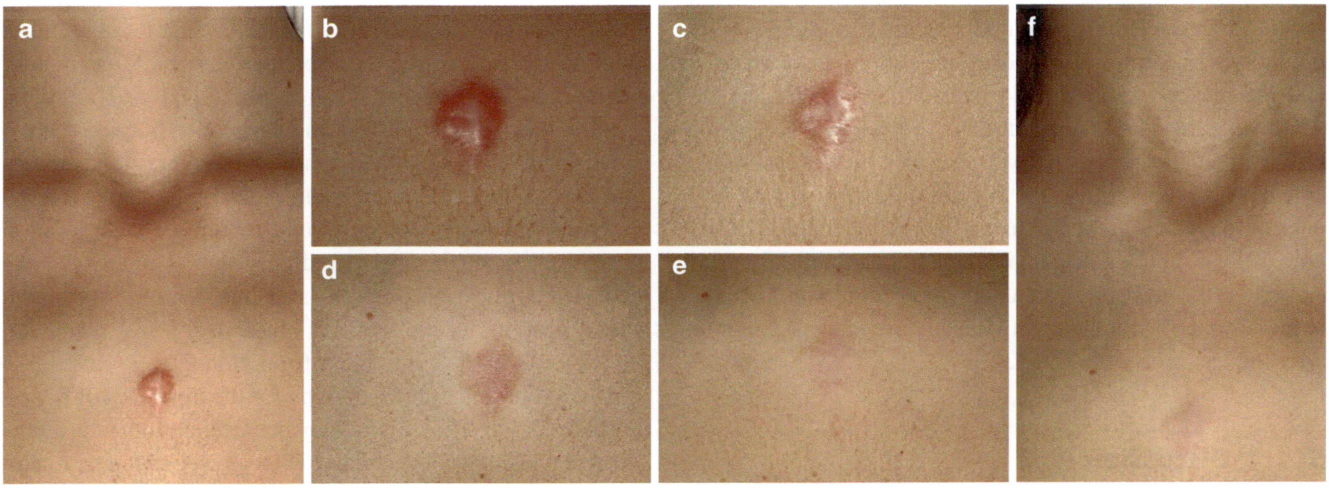

Fig. 1 Baseline photograph at presentation in our scar clinic before initiation of combination therapy with cryotherapy directly followed by intralesional TAC (**a**, **b**). Result after three cycles of combined cryo/intralesional TAC therapy before initiation of PDL (**c**). Result after four PDL applications and continuous administration of silicone gel demonstrating marked improvement of height and color (**d**). No signs of recurrence or reactivation at follow-up 6 months after the last laser treatment (**e**, **f**). Adapted from Clin Cosmet Investig Dermatol. 2013 Apr 24;6:103–14 [13]

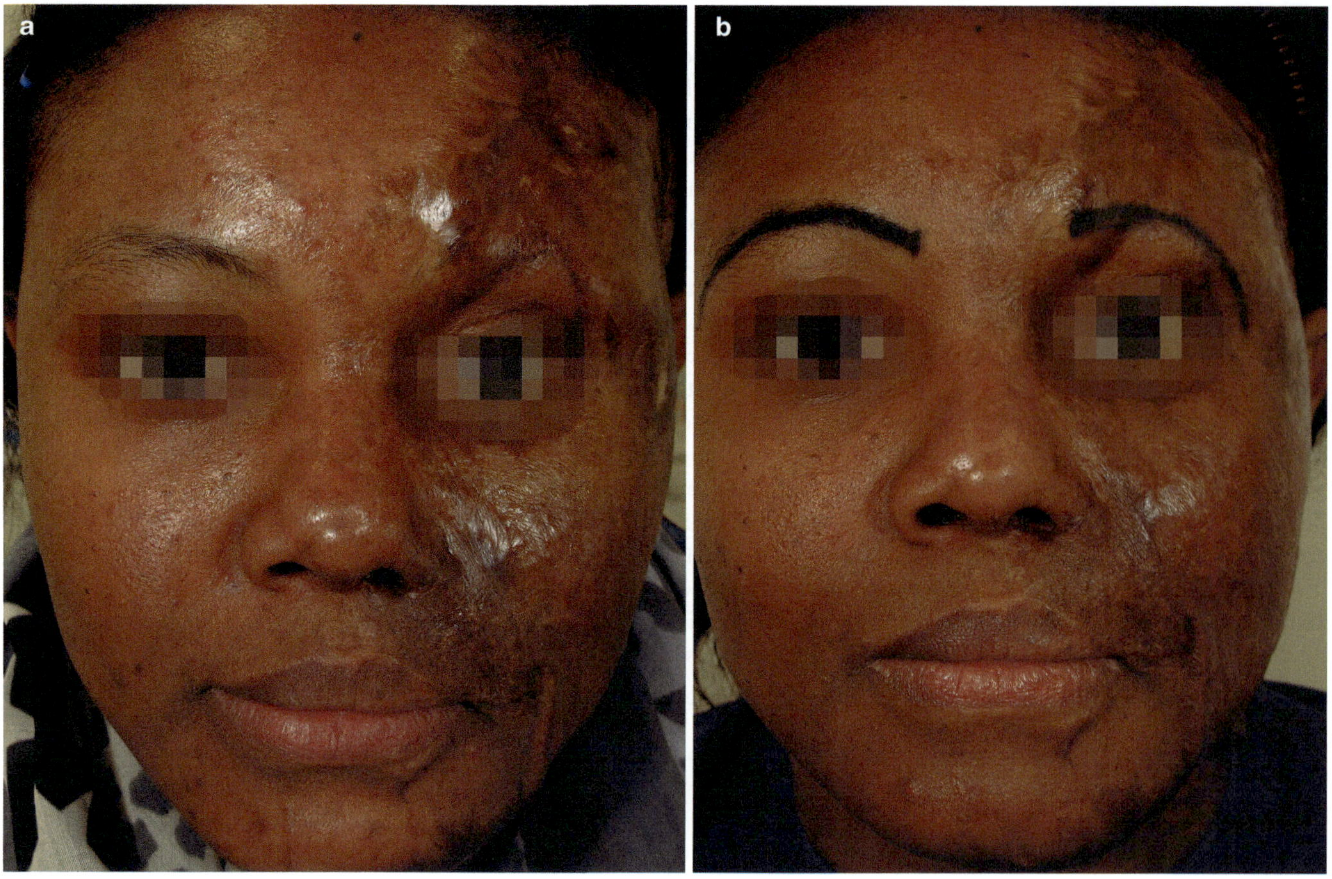

Fig. 2 Before (**a**) and after (**b**) 2x fractional CO_2 laser therapy (Scaar FX 70–110 mJ, Density 1%; Active FX, 2 passes; UltraPulse, Lumenis). With permission from JOURNAL OF WOUND TECHNOLOGY _ N° 31 _ JANUARY 2016

hyperpigmentation. However, the procedure was tolerated well thus treatment was initiated. Under local anesthesia cream for 1 h (Pliaglis, Galderma) and 1 g of paracetamol, the procedure was performed in three distinct steps. First, in order to introduce the scar remodeling process, the Scaar FX modality was employed with energies ranging in between 70 and 110 mJ/cm^2, 250 Hz, and a density of 1%. Next, the elevated scar areas were ablated using the Active FX technology with small spot sizes, lower energies (60–100 mJ/cm^2), and high densities. Last, the overall area was treated with another pass of Active FX using energies of 100–125 mJ/cm^2, 125 Hz, and a moderate density in an attempt to overall smoothen the respective area. This procedure was repeated twice around 3 months apart. Results are shown 3 months after the last procedure (Fig. 2b).

5 Discussion

Modern laser technology offers many safe and efficacious options for the treatment of hypertrophic scars and keloids to the trained practitioner. Able to improve both symptoms and aesthetically and functionally impairing scar parameters, the use of lasers for scar treatment can help to greatly improve the patients' well-being.

While mostly complementing conservative treatment options today, the future role of lasers in scar therapy might prove more vital. Through its potential in regard to symptom control and the improvement of functional and aesthetic impairments, laser treatment and especially fractional ablative resurfacing have gained a more important role in current guidelines and the recommendations of different expert committees. This might not only lead to further incorporation into future scar therapy paradigms but also lead to the increased application of early laser intervention to improve wound healing during the early phase of the scar formation process or to battle contracture formation [30].

The future role of laser therapy for the treatment of hypertrophic scars and keloids is, however, reliant on future prospective and controlled research. Since responsible treatment is both efficacious and safe while offering the treating physician maximum control throughout the treatment, a focus in future research has to be put on treatment methodology and finding the optimum laser settings for each indication.

References

1. Nast A, Eming S, Fluhr J, Fritz K, Gauglitz G, Hohenleutner S, et al. German S2k guidelines for the therapy of pathological scars (hypertrophic scars and keloids). J German Soc Dermatol. 2012;10(10):747–62.
2. Alster TS, Williams CM. Treatment of keloid sternotomy scars with 585 nm flashlamp-pumped pulsed-dye laser. Lancet. 1995;345(8959):1198–200.
3. Kuo YR, Wu WS, Jeng SF, Huang HC, Yang KD, Sacks JM, et al. Activation of ERK and p38 kinase mediated keloid fibroblast apoptosis after flashlamp pulsed-dye laser treatment. Lasers Surg Med. 2005;36(1):31–7.
4. Kuo YR, Wu WS, Jeng SF, Wang FS, Huang HC, Lin CZ, et al. Suppressed TGF-beta1 expression is correlated with up-regulation of matrix metalloproteinase-13 in keloid regression after flashlamp pulsed-dye laser treatment. Lasers Surg Med. 2005;36(1):38–42.
5. Tanzi EL, Alster TS. Laser treatment of scars. Skin Ther Lett. 2004;9(1):4–7.
6. Alster TS, Handrick C. Laser treatment of hypertrophic scars, keloids, and striae. Semin Cutan Med Surg. 2000;19(4):287–92.
7. Paquet P, Hermanns JF, Pierard GE. Effect of the 585 nm flashlamp-pumped pulsed dye laser for the treatment of keloids. Dermatol Surg. 2001;27(2):171–4.
8. Allison KP, Kiernan MN, Waters RA, Clement RM. Pulsed dye laser treatment of burn scars. Alleviation or irritation? Burns. 2003;29(3):207–13.
9. Wittenberg GP, Fabian BG, Bogomilsky JL, Schultz LR, Rudner EJ, Chaffins ML, et al. Prospective, single-blind, randomized, controlled study to assess the efficacy of the 585-nm flashlamp-pumped pulsed-dye laser and silicone gel sheeting in hypertrophic scar treatment. Arch Dermatol. 1999;135(9):1049–55.
10. Durani P, Bayat A. Levels of evidence for the treatment of keloid disease. J Plast Reconstr Aesthet Surg. 2008;61(1):4–17.
11. Alster T. Laser scar revision: comparison study of 585-nm pulsed dye laser with and without intralesional corticosteroids. Dermatol Surg. 2003;29(1):25–9.
12. Vrijman C, van Drooge AM, Limpens J, Bos JD, van der Veen JP, Spuls PI, et al. Laser and intense pulsed light therapy for the treatment of hypertrophic scars: a systematic review. Br J Dermatol. 2011;165(5):934–42.
13. Gauglitz GG. Management of keloids and hypertrophic scars: current and emerging options. Clin Cosmet Investig Dermatol. 2013;6:103–14.
14. Gold MH, Berman B, Clementoni MT, Gauglitz GG, Nahai F, Murcia C. Updated international clinical recommendations on scar management: part 1-evaluating the evidence. Dermatol Surg. 2014;40(8):817–24.
15. Gold MH, McGuire M, Mustoe TA, Pusic A, Sachdev M, Waibel J, et al. Updated international clinical recommendations on scar management: part 2-algorithms for scar prevention and treatment. Dermatol Surg. 2014;40(8):825–31.
16. Nouri K, Jimenez GP, Harrison-Balestra C, Elgart GW. 585-nm pulsed dye laser in the treatment of surgical scars starting on the suture removal day. Dermatol Surg. 2003;29(1):65–73; discussion.
17. Nouri K, Rivas MP, Stevens M, Ballard CJ, Singer L, Ma F, et al. Comparison of the effectiveness of the pulsed dye laser 585 nm versus 595 nm in the treatment of new surgical scars. Lasers Med Sci. 2009;24(5):801–10.
18. Cho SB, Lee JH, Lee SH, Lee SJ, Bang D, Oh SH. Efficacy and safety of 1064-nm Q-switched Nd:YAG laser with low fluence for keloids and hypertrophic scars. J Eur Acad Dermatol Venereol. 2010;24(9):1070–4.
19. Koike S, Akaishi S, Nagashima Y, Dohi T, Hyakusoku H, Ogawa R. Nd:YAG laser treatment for keloids and hypertrophic scars: an analysis of 102 cases. Plast Reconstr Surg Glob Open. 2014;2(12):e272.
20. Rossi A, Lu R, Frey MK, Kubota T, Smith LA, Perez M. The use of the 300 microsecond 1064 nm Nd:YAG laser in the treatment of keloids. J Drugs Dermatol. 2013;12(11):1256–62.
21. Dams SD, de Liefde-van Beest M, Nuijs AM, Oomens CW, Baaijens FP. Pulsed heat shocks enhance procollagen type I and procollagen type III expression in human dermal fibroblasts. Skin Res Technol. 2010;16(3):354–64.
22. Helbig D, Paasch U. Molecular changes during skin aging and wound healing after fractional ablative photothermolysis. Skin Res Technol. 2011;17(1):119–28.
23. Kwan JM, Wyatt M, Uebelhoer NS, Pyo J, Shumaker PR. Functional improvement after ablative fractional laser treatment of a scar contracture. PM & R. 2011;3(10):986–7.
24. Oh GAH, Choi JE, et al. Postoperative treatment of surgical scars with ablative fractional laser versus pulsed dye laser: a randomized controlled trial. J Am Acad Dermatol. 2012;66(4 Supplement 1):AB12.
25. Tierney E, Mahmoud BH, Srivastava D, Ozog D, Kouba DJ. Treatment of surgical scars with nonablative fractional laser versus pulsed dye laser: a randomized controlled trial. Dermatol Surg. 2009;35(8):1172–80.
26. Cervelli V, Gentile P, Spallone D, Nicoli F, Verardi S, Petrocelli M, et al. Ultrapulsed fractional CO2 laser for the treatment of post-traumatic and pathological scars. J Drugs Dermatol. 2010;9(11):1328–31.
27. Qu L, Liu A, Zhou L, He C, Grossman PH, Moy RL, et al. Clinical and molecular effects on mature burn scars after treatment with a fractional CO(2) laser. Lasers Surg Med. 2012;44(7):517–24.
28. Ozog DM, Liu A, Chaffins ML, Ormsby AH, Fincher EF, Chipps LK, et al. Evaluation of clinical results, histological architecture, and collagen expression following treatment of mature burn scars with a fractional carbon dioxide laser. JAMA Dermatol. 2013;149(1):50–7.
29. Suh D-H CK-Y, Song K-Y, et al. Revision of burn scars using ablative fractional CO_2 laser. J Am Acad Dermatol. 2012;66(4):AB216.
30. Anderson RR, Donelan MB, Hivnor C, Greeson E, Ross EV, Shumaker PR, et al. Laser treatment of traumatic scars with an emphasis on ablative fractional laser resurfacing: consensus report. JAMA Dermatol. 2014;150(2):187–93.

'Acid Attack' Scars: Strategy for Scars from Assaults Using Corrosive Substances

Kayvan Shokrollahi

The use of corrosive substances has unfortunately increased in some parts of the world including the UK; In 2006–2007, there were 44 admissions to hospital as a result of these assaults and there has been a year-on-year rise to 110 in 2010–2011. Recent evidence has shown that these attacks tend to occur in certain pockets of the country, mainly in the South East, that the victims tend to be Caucasian men and the perpetrators tend also to be Caucasian men. This is a previously undocumented demographic pattern.

The face is affected in 37% of such patients, followed by upper limb (23%), neck (16%), and the rest trunk and lower limb. Eye involvement is present in 43%.

Scarring and other problems as a result of these injuries manifest in a number of ways and often affects the face (Fig. 1a, b). Laser may be brought to bear to assist in some aspects of treatment of these scars, including:

- Scar folliculitis
- Heterotopic hair growth as a result of reconstructive surgery
- Pigmentary problems
- Atrophic scarring
- Hypertrophic and keloid scarring

1 Scar Folliculitis and Hair Removal

The use of lasers for depilation is well recognised. The most useful lasers include the alexandrite 755 nm wavelength long pulse laser, infrared diode lasers, and Nd:YAG lasers especially for darker skin types and for deeper hair in thicker scars.

The most severe types of scar folliculitis occur in skin types V–VI, and laser depilation is not typically useful in these severe cases, and new strategies are required.

K. Shokrollahi (✉)
Burns and Plastic Surgery Unit, Whiston Hospital, Liverpool, UK

Reconstructive surgery such as full-thickness skin grafts can often produce atypical hair-bearing areas on the face.

The symptomatic relief from successful laser treatment of scar folliculitis is difficult to quantify, nor is it easy to demonstrate visibly. However, it can be one of the most significant and impactful treatments delivered to this patient group and should always be discussed and offered as many patients may not be aware of its availability or utility.

2 Erythema and Hypertrophic Scars

Vascular lasers such as the pulsed dye laser (PDL), at wavelength 595 nm, or a long-pulsed Nd: YAG laser, wavelength 1064 nm, have the best evidence base for the treatment of scar erythema (Fig. 2), particularly hypertrophic scars. The greater depth of penetration in areas of thickened scarring may benefit from a combination of the two lasers, and some vascular laser systems have both lasers available 'in one box'.

3 Pigmentation

Carbon dioxide and Q-switched Nd:YAG lasers provide the mainstay of treatment for hyperpigmentation, but hypopigmentation has limited potential for improvement except cosmetic camouflage. Test patching with a range of Q-switched lasers and the carbon dioxide laser is the best starting point to ascertain efficacy.

4 Keloid Scars

Treatment of keloid scaring is especially challenging and typically requires a multimodal approach. Concurrent treatment using intralesional steroid injections and pressure garments or pressure masks is typically necessary, and it is

K. Shokrollahi (ed.), *Laser Management of Scars*, https://doi.org/10.1007/978-3-030-52919-2_12

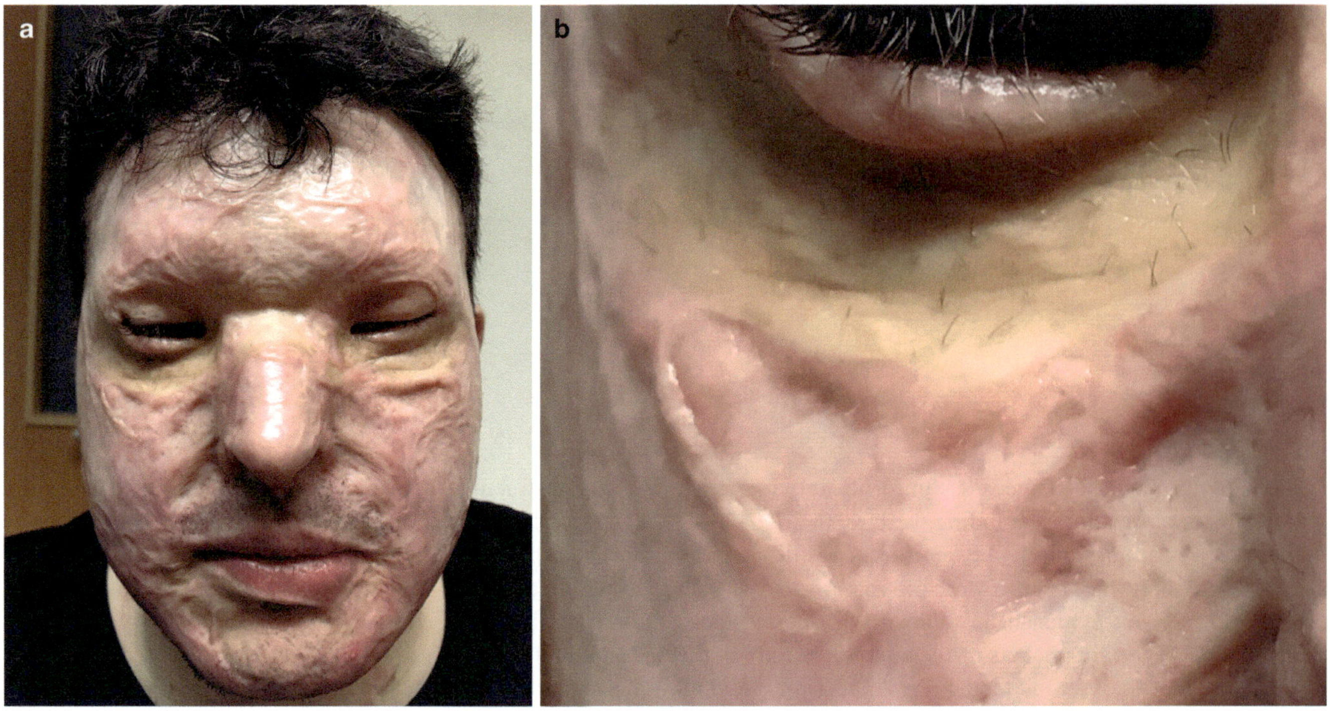

Fig. 1 (**a**) Thick hypertrophic scars with scar folliculitis in hair-bearing areas, along with scar erythema and contour issues. (**b**) Close up showing heterotopic hair of the lower eyelid from full-thickness skin grafts

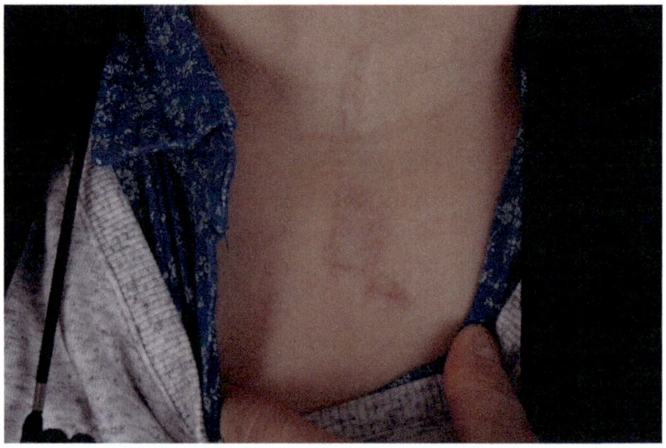

Fig. 2 Scar erythema with hypertrophic edges in a 'flow and drip' pattern after an acid attack

unlikely for keloid scarring to be successfully treated in the presence of any underlying scar folliculitis. Surgery is most often successful in circumstances where there has been delayed healing or infection during the healing process in skin that otherwise tends to heal without keloid scarring. The ancillary use of lasers may be helpful as follows:

- Treatment of the consequences of steroid injection, such as telangiectasia.
- Laser hair removal.
- Fractional laser resurfacing after extensive test patching, and possibly as a manner of therapeutic drug delivery which is a technique in its infancy. Ablative lasers must be used with extreme caution in patients with a tendency to develop keloid scars.
- Ablative 'intralesional' treatments to debulk scarring.
- Vascular lasers for erythema.

5 Atrophic Scars

Deep atrophic scarring (Fig. 3) is difficult to treat, unlike more superficial atrophic scarring that camouflages easily. The main options are surgery and thicker cosmetic camouflage including topical silicone fillers.

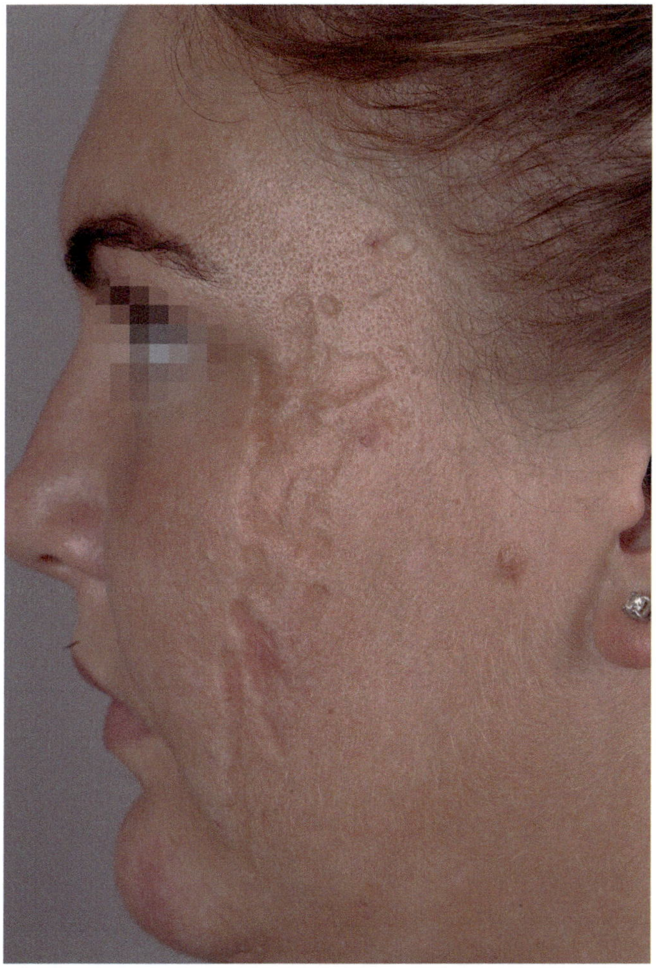

Fig. 3 Deep atrophic acid attack scar, part of which was subsequently surgically excised

Further Reading

1. Tan A, Bharj AK, Nizamoglu M, Barnes D, Dziewulski P. Assaults from corrosive substances and medico legal considerations in a large regional burn centre in the United Kingdom: calls for increased vigilance and enforced legislation. Scars burn heal. 2015;1:2059513115612945. https://doi.org/10.1177/2059513115612945.
2. Whiatker IS, Shokrollahi K, Dickson WA. Oxford Specialist Handbooks in Surgery: Burns 2019. Ch 9, Chemical Burns.
3. Shokrollahi K. Perspectives on acid attacks in the UK. Scars Burns Heal. 2017;3:2059513117723769. https://doi.org/10.1177/2059513117723769.

Photodynamic Therapy for the Treatment of Scars

Kayvan Shokrollahi and Charlotte Hardman

Photodynamic therapy (PDT) involves the use of a photosensitiser, a light source and the presence of oxygen to create reactive oxygen species (ROS) intercellularly. The accumulation of free radicals directs cell apoptosis and modulates cellular protein expression and signalling. PDT has a range of applications including treatment of cancers, in particular of the skin. It is recommended by the British Association of Dermatologist for actinic keratoses, Bowen's disease and superficial basal cell carcinoma [1]. Off label, it is used in inflammatory and infective conditions such as acne, psoriasis and viral warts [1, 2]. Recent research has found PDT to be effective in scar management including hypertrophic, keloid, striae and burns scars in animal, ex vivo and case studies. It is on this topic that this chapter focuses.

Over the last few decades, there have been a large number of natural and synthetic photosensitisers developed which can broadly be divided into porphyrins, chlorins and dyes. For dermatological indication, porphyrins photosensitisers are used, the main topical prodrug for which is 5-aminolevulinate acid (ALA) and its methyl ester form methyl aminolevulinate (MAL). ALA and MAL are synthesized in mitochondria and enter the porphyrin-heme pathway. They are converted through porphyrin intermediates in the cytosol into protoporphyrin IX (PpIX). PpIX is the active photosensitiser in PDT treatment. These prodrugs have a low molecular weight and thus can penetrate the stratum corneum. MAL being lipophilic has an enhanced penetration over ALA, although requires endogenous demethylation back to the non-ester form. In keloid fibroblasts, higher concentrations of PpIX were synthesized by equivalent dosages of MAL than by ALA. In the same study, ALA induced more PpIX accumulation in normal skin fibroblasts compared to MAL [3].

K. Shokrollahi (✉)
Burns and Plastic Surgery Unit, Whiston Hospital, Liverpool, UK

C. Hardman
Mersey Regional Centre for Burns and Plastic Surgery, Whiston Hospital, Liverpool, UK

When the photosensitizer PpIX is exposed to the visible light spectrum, ROS are generated. This occurs maximally at wavelengths 400–410 (blue) and 632–635 (red). PpIX will continue to be converted to heme to complete the porphyrin-heme pathway in mitochondria. Thus, maximum concentration of PpIX is between 4 and 6 h after the 3–4-h incubation of ALA/MAL topical application and is cleared between 24 and 50 h after application [4]. MAL-synthesized PpIX has been shown to disintegrate faster that ALA, (over 12 h) [3]. ALA is available as a 20% solution, MAL as a 16.8% cream [2].

ALA and MAL are thought to preferentially target epithelial tumours because of the cell's defective epidermal barrier and slower conversion of PpIX to heme [2]. They are preferentially absorbed by highly vascular or metabolically active tissue [5], which may be a relevant scar treatment. Yet, the precise mechanisms PDT improves scar outcomes are as yet not fully understood. Mills et al. [6] present the effects of PDT in normal wound healing, which provide important insights into the biochemical changes, that may explain PDT efficacy in scarred tissues. In their study, a 4-mm punch biopsy wound was created in skin and treated with MAL-PDT three times over 5 days. An identical control wound was untreated and both wounds left to heal by secondary intention. Wounds were re-excised during the inflammatory phase, matrix remodelling and final dermal structure (7 days, 3 weeks, 9 months consecutively). MAL-PDT delayed re-epithelialization at 7 days, but increased matrix metalloproteinase (MMP), MMP-1, MMP-9 and TGF-β3 production during matrix remodelling. At 9 months, these scars had an improved dermal matrix architecture with more ordered deposition of collagen I, collagen III and elastin.

In pathological scarring, PDT has been shown to target diseased tissue [7, 8] and may act on keratinocytes and fibroblasts or directly on collagen and extracellular matrixes in tissues: modulating growth factors, cytokines, transcription factors and metalloproteinases [9]. Part of the challenge to understanding the cellular mechanism of PDT in improved

K. Shokrollahi (ed.), *Laser Management of Scars*, https://doi.org/10.1007/978-3-030-52919-2_13

pathological scarring is the lack of understanding over the development of pathological skin healing itself.

As many scars are treated with excision, there are several studies examining the effect of PDT on these ex vivo scar samples. The majority of this research focuses on keloid [3, 10–14] and hypertrophic scaring [10, 15, 17, 18] but striae [10, 19] has also been considered. Evidence of PDT as effective and acceptable treatment for scars is building. The majority of in vivo cases show significant scar improvement in both keloid [5, 8, 20–22] and hypertrophic scarring [23–25] as well evidence from specific scarring sequelae such as from burns [25] and a case from scars post lupus miliaris [26]. The side effect profile of treatment has been found to be acceptable [8, 9].

1 Keloid Ex Vivo Studies

In keloid fibroblastic cells, PDT has significant association with increased levels of ROS, cell apoptosis and inhibition of cell proliferation. Jiao et al. [11] has shown a dose-dependant relationship with PDT treatment and fibroblasts inhibition from keloid scar tissue. Here, cells were incubated in vitro in 0, 1, 3, 6 and 9 mmol/L ALA. Then they were exposed to 635 nm wavelength red light (30 J/cm^2). The inhibition rate of keloid fibroblasts in respect to the increasing concentrations of ALA were 0, 8, 29, 52 and 80%. The content of hydroxyproline (a major component of collagen) inversely correlated with ALA concentration at: 10, 6, 5, 3.5 and 2.9 μg/mg. The difference was statistically significant when comparing treated verses non-treated groups ($P < 0.05$).

Mendoza-Garcia and the Manchester-based research group looked at PDT in keloid scar tissue was embedded in rat-tail collagen I and treated with PDT (632 nm, 37 J/cm^2), after application of ALA or MAL and incubation for 3 h [7]. They showed a tissue depth related cytotoxicity decreased from the epidermis to the inner reticular dermal layers of the keloid tissue. Penetration depth is a known limiting factor for thick keloid scars as ALA and MAL penetrate approximating 3 mm [1]. In addition to necrotic and apoptotic mechanisms causing decreased cellularity, an increased expression of caspases and MMP was observed in this study [7]. Further research in 2015 [10], immunohistochemically quantified 18 samples of striae alba, fine line, hypertrophic and keloid scars ex vivo after an equivalent photodynamic therapy. Again, after treatment apoptosis increased, which correlated with decreased cell proliferation along with proliferating cell nuclear antigen (PCNA) gene expression. Matrix components were found to be re-organized in both hypertrophic and keloid scars. Collagens I and III gene expression levels decreased, whilst MMP-3 and tropoelastin increased significantly post-PDT compared to normal skin and untreated controls ($P < 0.05$). The morphological and cellular effect of PDT were found to correlate with the degree and severity of dermal fibrosis; in view of this, PDT appears to be effective at naturally targeting treatment to abnormally scarred skin.

Zheng et al. [12] found that Runt-related transcription factor 3 (RUNX3) expression was detected more often in keloid tissues than in dermis of normal skin and was also significantly related to PCNA expression. Additionally, RUNX3 expression was significantly increased in symptomatic keloid scars—those with symptoms of pain or pruritus. Post-PDT significant differences were found between keloid fibroblasts with and without RUNX3 expression in generation of ROS, cell viability, apoptosis, proliferative ability and type I collagen expression. Thus, RUNX3 is a possible contributor to keloid pathogenesis and may improve keloid fibroblast sensitivity to PDT.

Mendoza et al. [13] investigated spatial relationship of PDT and cellular effect. ALA and MAL were applied to keloid fibroblasts from different lesional scar sites (top, middle and margin) ($n = 8$) and compared to normal skin fibroblasts ($n = 3$). PpIX accumulation was higher in fibroblasts from middle of the keloid as compared to cells from other sites which adds to the theory that PDT correlates with the degree and severity of dermal fibrosis and thus effectively targets scarred tissue. Fluorescence analysis in the same study revealed ROS-mediated cytotoxicity was light energy dependent. MAL instigated higher keloid fibroblast cytotoxicity at lower fluence (≤ 20 J/cm^2) while ALA instigated higher keloid fibroblast cytotoxicity at higher fluence, except in cells derived from the middle of the keloid. Senescence was not observed at higher light energies (>10 J/cm^2). The idea of senescence is not explored significantly in the paper, but Blazic et al. [14] present a related hypothesis: senescent fibroblasts form during wound repair, as the result of oxidative stress. They act as inhibitors in the control of fibroblast proliferation and extracellular matrix synthesis. The defective induction of stress-induced senescent phenotype creates an insufficient number of senescent cells and thus may relate to the uncontrolled hyperproliferation in keloid formation. The concept would be that grading PDT treatment to produce sublethal doses could cause senescence instead of cell death and this may improve outcome. This has yet to be substantiated, but an interesting concept when considering PDT dosage. Dosage and cell necrosis are explored in the study on hypertrophic scarring by Xin et al. [15].

Ex vivo keloid results have also shown significance when PDT is used in combination with other treatment modalities. The addition of electrical waveform stimulation in combination with PDT [3] has shown a significant increase compared to PDT alone across measures of cytotoxicity of keloid fibroblasts, ROS generation, apoptosis by caspase-3 activation, mitochondrial membrane depolarization and collagens I and III gene downregulation. There was no significant difference in the cytotoxicity of normal skin fibroblasts after any treatment (combined or singular). The electrical stimulation used was of a non-invasive electrical stimulation, a degenerate sine waveform based on the Fenzian electrical biofeedback system. This is one of the several electrical stimulation subtypes that have been shown to be effective in enhancing cutaneous wound healing [16].

2 Hypertrophic Ex Vivo Studies

In an ex vivo study on five hypertrophic scar samples, fibroblasts were isolated and treated with ALA-PDT [17]. PpIX accumulation peak was achieved at 1.0 mM ALA. Range 0–1.0 mM was demonstrated to be non-cytotoxic but reduced cell viabilities in a dose-dependent manner. Reduction of cell viability was attributed mainly to cell apoptosis and probably to mechanisms such as upregulation of p53/p21, Bax/Bcl-2 ratio and cleaved caspase-3. Transforming growth factor-β1-mediated signalling, which has been proposed as a mechanism underlying hypertrophic scar formation, was found to be reversely modulated in response to therapy. These results were consistent with another study on five hypertrophic scar samples which were compared to normal controls [17]. Hypertrophic scar–derived fibroblasts were found to efficiently accumulate PpIX after ALA treatment, which caused cell apoptosis in a dose-dependent manner with energy density. Here, apoptotic cell death was observed with low-dose PDT, whereas necrotic cells were increased by high-dose PDT. Treatment was with 5 h of ALA treatment at 1 mmol/L concentration, 635 nm wavelength laser (red) at a power density of 10 mW/cm^2, with an energy density from 0.5 to 4 J/cm^2. At 4 J/cm^2 40% of fibroblasts had undergone necrosis, whilst this was only 6% at 3 J/cm^2. Zhong et al. [18] also sort to determine the effect of ALA-PDT on fibroblast cells from hypertrophic scars in vitro and to identify proper dosage of photosensitizer and energy level of laser light. Results showed the inhibition rate increased with the dosage of photosensitizer and the energy level of laser light. Maximal inhibition effect reached with 20 J/cm^2 laser light exposure and 0.5 mmol/L of ALA. These ex vivo dosage regimes need further application to in vivo studies to appreciate dosage efficacy and side effects.

PDT treatment for striae distensae scarring was considered in the 2015 study by Mendoza [10] as already discussed. The same research group sort to assess the effects of PDT on striae distensae skin in isolation [19]. Striae alba tissue ($n = 4$) was embedded in rat-tail collagen I and treated with PDT-ALA or MAL for 2 h and followed by illumination with red light (632 nm) at 10 or 37 J/cm^2. Histological evaluation was performed day 7 post-treatment. Epidermal rearrangement was observed post-PDT at 10 J/cm^2 as well as loosening of papillary dermis with no apparent alteration of the basement membrane or reticular dermis. Total separation of the epidermal layer from the dermis was observed post-PDT at 37 J/cm^2. MAL had more significant effects on the tissue compared to ALA; an increased expression of elastin and MMPs was observed in addition to the decreased expression of collagen I. The study represents preliminary histological evidence that low energy doses of PDT may also improve the appearance of striae distensae.

3 Evidence for PDT in Keloid Scarring

In the review by Mamalis et al. [5], three papers on PDT in keloid treatment were found, which all showed improved scar outcomes. A case study found five treatments of MAL-PDT to a recurrent keloid resulted in a reduction in size, volume and erythema, with no recurrence at 1-year follow-up [20]. Ud-din et al. [8] described results from a case series of 20 patients, who received three weekly treatments of MAL-PDT. The regime was based on that used in this case study described [20]; MAL topical application for 3 h followed by irradiation at a 630 nm wavelength and light dosage was administered at 37 J/cm^2. Clinically improvements in pruritus, pain and pliability were found across the cases post-treatment [8]. Collagen levels ($p = 0.066$), haemoglobin levels ($p = 0.060$) and the mean blood flow in the area treated ($p = 0.032$) (measured in haemoglobin flux) decreased from week 1 to 3 in all except one patient (95%). Increases in pliability were significantly related to decreases in flux ($p = 0.001$). One patient with a keloid in a stress-prone anatomical location experienced recurrence of keloid disease (5%). No other cases were found to have recurrence at 9-month follow-up.

The Mamalis review considered penetration depth to be a potential limit to efficacy and suggested studies on combined treatments. The results of the Ud-din study were based on keloid scars that had no more than a 2 mm thickness (ten cases), those thicker were included as a post-surgical debulked scar (keloid scars of any size reduced/debulked to a keloid scar of at most a height of 2 mm) (six cases) or a post-total surgical excision (of any size scar which was removed in total) (four cases). Thus, these results need to be understood as PDT treatment for "thin" keloid scarring and as PDT as an adjuvant treatment to surgical debulking/excision for keloid scarring. Excision is quite a standard initial step for keloid scar management, followed by treatment to reduced recurrence, but it is important to appreciate thick PDT treatment will require initial surgical management.

Basdew et al. [21] looked the effectiveness of adjuvant PDT after keloid excision, but with a comparison group of keloid excision followed by brachytherapy. Forty-five keloids in 34 patients were evaluated using the Patient and Observer Scar Assessment Scale (POSAS) and no quantitative data was collected. Twenty-seven lesions received brachytherapy and 18 lesions received PDT. The observers scored a mean POSAS of 19.1 (range 13.0–34.0) for brachytherapy and 24.6 (range 11.0–37.0) for PDT ($p = 0.005$). The patients reported a significantly better mean POSAS score after brachytherapy (22.8, range 7.0–53.0) than following PDT (34.2, range 11.0–63.0). Patients and observers appeared to be more satisfied with the results after brachytherapy than PDT. Nonetheless, patients still have a positive general impression after PDT.

In a more specific indication: two cases of earlobe keloids after a piercing were treated with intralesional photodynamic therapy with good results [22]. Both had been previously treated with topical treatments, IPL and intralesional steroids without success. Here 1% lyophilized 5-aminolevulinic acid (dissolved into a saline solution) was injected inside the lesion, incubated for 2 h and then irradiated using a diode laser beam of 630 nm. In one case, the light source was applied intratumorally with a fibre-optic probe, while it was treated externally with the same light source. Patients needed two to three sessions to achieve the results of decrease scar size and disappearance of symptoms. After a follow-up of almost 2 years, neither case had recurred.

4 Evidence for PDT in Hypertrophic Scarring

The case for PDT in hypertrophic scars has also been building. In 2011, Bruscino et al. [23] describe a 69-year-old female who had a hypertrophic scarring on the right cheek due to a dog bite injury. She had failed treatment with topical and intralesional treatments. MAL-PDT with red light (wavelength of 632 nm) was repeated four times at 2-week intervals. Results at a month were a significantly softened, flexible and smoother scar with less erythematous and reduced volume. The was no recurrence at 1-year follow-up.

Fang et al. [24] looked at PDT as an adjuvant treatment to steroid injection. Thirty-seven cases of hypertrophic scarring were divided into case control groups. The treatment was found effective in 55.6% of the steroid control group ($n = 18$), compared to 89.5% in the steroid and PDT group ($n = 19$) ($P = 0.029$). Additionally, the recurrence rate in treatment group was also significantly lower than that in the control group ($P = 0.047$).

The results of two patients with significant hypertrophic scaring as a result of burns injury are presented by Cambell et al. [25]. The first case was a 42-year-old man with extensive hypertrophic scarring and contractures across his chest as a result of thermal burns as a child. His main symptoms were of tightness causing splitting and pain on expansion of the chest wall. The second case was a female with thickened hypertrophic scarring in the right axilla after burn injury. Metvix® (MAL) 16.8% cream was applied to the area 1 mm thick and occluded with a light resistant dressing for 4 h. Light was applied using a Aktilite® light source at 37 J/cm^2, 635 ± 2 nm. Results were studied by fluorescence imaging throughout the treatment and by histological samples (punch biopsies) taken pre and 6 weeks post-treatment. The fluorescence images showed PpIX accumulation in the scarred tissue after MAL application, followed by a return to baseline levels immediately following light irradiation. Clinically, the scarred areas had significantly softened and become more flexible as judged by pinching the skin. Ulceration had settled and scar discomfort was reduced.

Histologically, pre-treatment biopsies show plate-like areas of collagen deposition in the mid and deep dermis. Superficially, there were reasonable numbers of elastic fibres present but these were almost absent in the thickened collagen scar. Fibroblasts could be seen cuffing the collagen. Results at 6 weeks showed a larger number of elastin fibres both within superficial and deep skin tissue sections.

A case of refractory lupus scarring treated with MAL-PDT was studied Borgia et al. [26]. The red-atrophic scars post Lupus miliaris disseminatus faciei achieved significant improvement after three sessions of ALA-PDT with 10% aminolevulinic acid. The results were considered to potentially be a consequence of the combined anti-inflammatory, immunomodulatory and keratinocytes activation.

None of the studies reported significant side effects. Ud-din et al. [8] found inflammation was reported by 15% (3/20) of cases, lasting an average of 2 days. Pigment changes were also noted by 15%, and these patients had a Fitzpatrick score of 3 or above.

5 Conclusion

The biochemical mechanisms by which PDT directs cell apoptosis and modulates cellular protein expression and signalling in pathological scarring states has been explored in ex vivo and in vivo models. ALA/MAL accumulates in pathologically scarred tissue including keloid, hypertrophic and striae scarring, and this accumulation increased with increasing dermal fibrosis. PDT exhibits a dose-related response both in concentration of photosensitizer and in light intensity which indicates validity of results viewed. After PDT treatment in keloid and hypertrophic scarring fibroblasts showed significantly increased levels of ROS, MMP-3, caspase-3 and tropoelastin. Upregulation of p53/p21, Bax/Bcl-2 ratio was also suggested. Collagens I and III gene expression levels decreased, along with proliferating cell nuclear antigen. These biochemical alterations directed cell apoptosis and inhibited cell proliferation. Matrix components were found to be re-organized in both hypertrophic and keloid scars, and hypertrophic scars were found to have larger number of elastin fibres post-PDT. Transforming growth factor-β1-mediated signalling, which has been proposed as a mechanism underlying hypertrophic scar formation, was found to be reversely modulated in response to therapy. RUNX3 was found to be a possible contributor to keloid pathogenesis and was seen to improve keloid fibroblast sensitivity to PDT.

Clinically, penetration is a known limiting factor for thick keloid scars, but in these cases adjuvant PDT post-scar debulking/excision had good results. In hypertrophic scarring tissue, modulation occurred in deep dermal tissue as well as superficial. Standard licenced concentrations of ALA/MAL were used in in vivo studies for obvious reasons. Rising concentrations of ALA ex vivo created a proportional inhibition rate of keloid fibroblasts. Energy density varied from study to study. In vivo up to 37 J/cm^2 was used, yet ex vivo studies suggested increased cell necrosis above 4 J/cm^2. The concept of graded PDT dosage to produce senescent fibroblasts instead of cell death was discussed as a theory that may improve outcome, but this has yet to be substantiated.

The most striking evidence for efficacy in scar management thus far for PDT is presented in the Ud-din study of 20 cases [8]. In thin keloid scarring and surgically excised keloid disease, recurrence rates after PDT were 5%, compared to the usual 50% post excision alone. Collagen, haemoglobin and mean blood flow decreased post-treatment. Pruritus, pain and pliability all improved. In hypertrophic scarring, impressive results were found concerning large surface area burns scars, with positive patient, observer and histological outcomes, nonetheless this was only in a case series of 2.

Overall case evidence is very much in its infancy. There is a lack of comparative studies and the only one, comparing brachy therapy, showed PDT to be less effective than brachy therapy, but without recourse to either surgery or ionizing radiation. Nonetheless, the case studies discussed which have shown significantly scar improvements histologically and as per observed and patient ratings certainly warrant larger studies in the field.

The role of PDT as a combined modality is yet to be explored; the review by Fang et al. [24] looked at PDT as an adjuvant treatment to steroid injection, which showed an improved outcome with combined therapy over steroid alone. There is certainly scope for more studies looking at the adjuvant outcomes of combined therapy with other modalities known to improve scar outcomes: such as silicon-based therapy, radiofrequency ablation, 5-fluorouracil and other forms of light therapy; intense pulsed light, fractional CO_2 laser and pulsed dye laser.

Lastly, PDT has a range of desirable attributes as a treatment for scarring including simplicity, accessibility, lack of ionizing radiation (compared to radiotherapy or brachy therapy) and treatment in an outpatient only setting. PDT is now used with daylight sensitisation for the treatment of actinic keratoses [27], and this has the potential for development in the management of scars; for example, the treatment of hypertrophic scarring on the face. This could further simplify treatment and reduce time in clinic. PDT does look to be a useful weapon in the armory against pathological scarring, and we shall eagerly await further studies on the subject.

Note on terminology. The recent Chinese guidelines on scar prevention and treatment highlight the value of photodynamic therapy for several aspects of scar management [28]. It is important to appreciate that 'photodynamic therapy' in that document appears to refer to laser and light source therapies and not photodynamic therapy in the true sense that requires a photosensitizer drugs.

References

1. Morton CA, McKenna KE, Rhodes LE. Guidelines for topical photodynamic therapy: update. Br J Dermatol. 2008;159(6):1245–66.
2. Ozog DM, Rkein AM, Fabi SG, Gold MH, Goldman MP, Lowe NJ, et al. Photodynamic therapy: a clinical consensus guide. Dermatol Surg. 2016;42:804–27.
3. Sebastian A, Allan E, Allan D, Colthurst J, Bayat A. Addition of novel degenerate electrical waveform stimulation with photodynamic therapy significantly enhances its cytotoxic effect in keloid fibroblasts: first report of a potential combination therapy. J Dermatol Sci. 2011;64(3):174–84.
4. Golub AL, Gudgin Dickson EF, Kennedy JC, Marcus SL, Park Y, Pottier RH. The monitoring of ALA-induced Protoporphyrin IX accumulation and clearance in patients with skin lesions by in vivo surface-detected fluorescence spectroscopy. Lasers Med Sci. 1999;14(2):112–22.
5. Mamalis AD, Lev-Tov H, Nguyen D-H, Jagdeo JR. Laser and light-based treatment of keloids--a review. J Eur Acad Dermatol Venereol. 2014;28(6):689–99.
6. Mills SJ, Farrar MD, Ashcroft GS, Griffiths CEM, Hardman MJ, Rhodes LE. Topical photodynamic therapy following excisional wounding of human skin increases production of transforming growth factor-beta3 and matrix metalloproteinases 1 and 9, with associated improvement in dermal matrix organization. Br J Dermatol. 2014;171(1):55–62.
7. Mendoza Garcia J, Alonso-Rasgado T, Bayat Sebastian A. EX vivo verification with histology of the effect of photodynamic therapy in reduction of keloid scar volume (conference abstract). Wound Repair Regen. 2013. May 2013. Wound Repair and Regeneration 21(2). Conference: 23rd annual meeting of the wound healing society with SAWC 2013, denver, colorado, USAAT: wound repair and regeneration. 2013;21(2):179–337, A13–A54.
8. Ud-Din S, Thomas G, Morris J, Bayat A. Photodynamic therapy: an innovative approach to the treatment of keloid disease evaluated using subjective and objective non-invasive tools. Arch Dermatol Res. 2013;305(3):205–14.
9. Nie Z. Is photodynamic therapy a solution for keloid? G Ital Dermatol Venereol. 2011;146(6):463–72.
10. Mendoza-Garcia J, Sebastian A, Alonso-Rasgado T, Bayat A. Ex vivo evaluation of the effect of photodynamic therapy on skin scars and striae distensae. Photodermatol Photoimmunol Photomed. 2015;31(5):239–51.
11. Jiao J, Fan Y. [Effect of photodynamic therapy on the cell proliferation and collagen secretion of keloid fibroblasts]. Zhonghua Zheng Xing Wai Ke Za Zhi. 2015;31(1):49–53.
12. Zheng Z, Zhu L, Zhang X, Li L, Moon S, Roh MR, et al. RUNX3 expression is associated with sensitivity to pheophor-

bide a-based photodynamic therapy in keloids. Lasers Med Sci. 2015;30(1):67–75.
13. Mendoza J, Sebastian A, Allan E, Allan D, Mandal P, Alonso-Rasgado T, et al. Differential cytotoxic response in keloid fibroblasts exposed to photodynamic therapy is dependent on photosensitiser precursor, fluence and location of fibroblasts within the lesion. Arch Dermatol Res. 2012;304(7):549–62.
14. Blazic TM, Brajac I. Defective induction of senescence during wound healing is a possible mechanism of keloid formation. Med Hypotheses. 2006;66(3):649–52.
15. Li X, Zhou ZP, Hu L, Zhang WJ, Li W. Apoptotic cell death induced by 5-aminolaevulinic acid-mediated photodynamic therapy of hypertrophic scar-derived fibroblasts. J Dermatolog Treat. 2014;25(5):428–33.
16. Petrofsky JS, Lawson D, Berk L, Suh H. Enhanced healing of diabetic foot ulcers using local heat and electrical stimulation for 30 min three times per week. J Diabetes. 2010;2(1):41–6.
17. Chang M, Ma X, Ouyang T, Lin J, Liu J, Xiao Y, et al. Potential molecular mechanisms involved in 5-aminolevulinic acid-based photodynamic therapy against human hypertrophic scars. Plast Reconstr Surg. 2015;136(4):715–27.
18. Zhong J-B, Wang L, Luo L-D, Pan L. [Influence of ALA-PDT on fibroblast cells from hypertrophic scars]. Sichuan Da Xue Xue Bao Yi Xue Ban. 2011;42(4):515–8.
19. Mendoza-Garcia J, Sebastian A, Alonso-Rasgado T, Bayat A. Ex vivo evaluation of the effect of photodynamic therapy on skin scars and striae distensae. Photodermatol Photoimmunol Photomed. 2015;31(5):239–51. https://doi.org/10.1111/phpp.12180.
20. Nie Z, Bayat A, Behzad F, Rhodes LE. Positive response of a recurrent keloid scar to topical methyl aminolevulinate-photodynamic therapy. Photodermatol Photoimmunol Photomed. 2010;26(6):330–2.
21. Besdew H, Mehilal R, Al-Mamgani A, van Rooji P, et al. Adjunctive treatment of keloids: comparison of photodynamic therapy with brachytherapy. Eur J Plast Surg. 2013;36(5):289–94.
22. Tosa M, Ogawa R. Photodynamic therapy for keloids and hypertrophic scars: a review. Scars Burn Heal. 2020;6:2059513120932059. https://doi.org/10.1177/2059513120932059. PMID: 32655901; PMCID: PMC7328485.
23. Bruscino N, Lotti T, Rossi R. Photodynamic therapy for a hypertrophic scarring: a promising choice. Photodermatol Photoimmunol Photomed. 2011;27(6):334–5.
24. Fang F, Hong Z, Yan Z, Meiling L. [Application of photodynamic therapy combined with compound betamethasone in treatment of hypertrophic scar]. Zhonghua Zheng Xing Wai Ke Za Zhi.2015;31(5):343–6.
25. Campbell SM, Tyrrell J, Marshall R, Curnow A. Effect of MAL-photodynamic therapy on hypertrophic scarring. Photodiagnosis Photodyn Ther. 2010;7(3):183–8.
26. Borgia F, Giuffrida R, Vaccaro M, Lentini M, Cannavo SP. Photodynamic therapy in lupus miliaris disseminatus faciei's scars. Dermatol Ther. 2016;29(5):320–4.
27. See J, Shumack S, Murrell DF, et al. Consensus recommendations on the use of daylight photodynamic therapy with methyl aminolevulinate cream for actinic keratoses in Australia. Australas J Dermatol. 2016;57(3):167–74. https://doi.org/10.1111/ajd.12354.
28. Lv K, Xia Z. Chinese expert consensus on clinical prevention and treatment of scar. Burn Trauma. 2018;6:27.

1550-nm Erbium:Glass and 1927-nm Thulium Non-Ablative Fractional Lasers for the Treatment of Burn Scars

Joy Tao, David Surprenant, Amanda Champlain, Charles Weddington, Lauren Moy, and Rebecca Tung

1 Introduction

Burn scars cause significant morbidity due to cosmetic disfigurement, contractures, associated symptoms such as pain and pruritus, and psychosocial distress [1]. Patients with burn scars often have a diminished quality of life, difficulties with social interactions, and frequently suffer from anxiety, depression, and low self-esteem [2]. While advancements in care have dramatically decreased mortality from burn injuries, the management of burn scars remains challenging [3, 4]. Numerous burn scars treatments exist, including silicone gel sheeting, scar massage therapy, compression garments, cryotherapy, corticosteroid injections, and surgical interventions. Regardless of therapeutic modality chosen, outcomes are variable [1].

The treatment of scars has evolved with the availability of fractional laser devices. Fractional resurfacing lasers insert hundreds of evenly distributed columns of thermal injury, referred to as microscopic treatment zones (MTZ), into the dermis [1, 5]. The pulse energy and treatment density determine the depth of injury and number of MTZs per treatment area, respectively [1]. At each session, fractional resurfacing lasers only treat a percentage of the cross-sectional area of skin [6]. Untreated skin between MTZs promotes rapid post-procedure healing and collagen remodeling [7]. Histopathologic changes seen in burn scars treated with fractional lasers include increased vascularity, decreased inflammation, and alteration of collagen. These histopathologic changes correlate with more normal appearing skin [8].

Ablative fractional lasers are frequently employed to treat burn scars. Ablative lasers work via targeted tissue destruction. While effective, their use is associated with prolonged downtime and an increased risk of extensive side effects, especially in patients with darker skin tones who are more prone to post-laser hyperpigmentation [9–11].

Non-ablative fractional lasers (NAFL) present a viable alternative in the treatment of burn scars in patients who desire a less aggressive, more gradual treatment approach [6]. Rather than vaporizing tissue, NAFL work by heating up targeted tissue and stimulating tissue remodeling in a much less-invasive manner.

2 Review of the Evidence

Non-ablative fractional resurfacing lasers have shown to be effective in improving thickness, pliability, pigmentary changes, and textural abnormalities in both early and mature scars [9]. These types of lasers include the 1550-nm erbium:glass laser and the 1927-nm thulium laser.

The 1550-nm wavelength erbium:glass laser has many applications including photoaging, rhytids, melasma, and other skin textural abnormalities [12]. This laser can also be used to improve the appearance and texture of various types of scars, including burn scars. Treatment with the 1550-nm wavelength laser improves burn scars by stimulating collagen remodeling through controlled dermal injury [13]. The majority of treated patients find improvement in scar texture, contracture, discoloration, atrophy, and hypertrophy. It should

Contents of Chapter originally printed in: *Scars, Burns & Healing*. *DOI:* https://doi.org/10.1177/2059513118758510
Tao J, Champlain A, Weddington C, Moy L, Tung R. Treatment of burn scars in Fitzpatrick phototype III patients with a combination of pulsed dye laser and non-ablative fractional resurfacing 1550 nm erbium:glass/1927 nm thulium laser devices. *Scars, Burns & Healing*. 2018;4:1–6. DOI: https://doi.org/10.1177/2059513118758510

J. Tao (✉) · D. Surprenant · A. Champlain · L. Moy
Division of Dermatology, Loyola University Chicago, Chicago, IL, USA
e-mail: jtao2@luc.edu; lauren.moy001@lumc.edu

C. Weddington
Department of Dermatology, University of Maryland, Baltimore, MD, USA
e-mail: cweddington@som.umaryland.edu

R. Tung
Florida Dermatology and Skin Cancer Centers, Winter Haven, FL, USA

K. Shokrollahi (ed.), *Laser Management of Scars*, https://doi.org/10.1007/978-3-030-52919-2_14

be noted that thinner scars tend to respond more favorably to treatment than bulkier, hypertrophic scars [1]. Treatment may also alleviate associated scar symptoms such as pain and pruritus [13, 14]. Overall, the 1550-nm erbium:glass laser has been found to be safe and effective with the advantage of less downtime when compared to ablative lasers.

The 1927-nm wavelength thulium laser can be utilized to improve both scar texture and associated post-inflammatory hyperpigmentation. The 1927-nm wavelength targets dyspigmentation by shuttling melanin into collections of microscopic necrotic debris just above MTZs. This epidermal debris is then subsequently shed after 1–2 weeks [7, 15]. The thulium laser is frequently used to treat various pigmentary disorders, such as melasma and post-inflammatory hyperpigmentation, with minimal side effects [16–21]. Additionally, several reports found that the thulium fractional laser can dramatically improve the appearance of photo-damaged–induced dyspigmentation, ephelides, lentigines, and keratosis [22–25].

The 1550-nm erbium and 1927-thulium laser are frequently used together to target photo-damaged skin and rhytids with no major adverse effects [26]. These lasers used in combination can also be employed to soften scars and improve scar laxity, helping minimize the range of motion limitations caused by scar contracture [14]. The 1550-nm erbium laser and 1927-nm thulium laser used in combination can significantly improve the texture and color of burn scars [27].

3 Treatment Methodology

Patients with mild-to-severe burn scars can be treated with the 1550-nm erbium:glass/1927-nm thulium dual wavelength laser device (Fraxel DUAL, Solta Medical, Hayward, CA). Patients who are especially concerned about prolonged downtime and adverse effects of more aggressive laser types and would prefer a more gentle treatment approach may benefit the most from these lasers. Patients with darker skin tones should be counseled on the increased risk of post-inflammatory hyperpigmentation (PIH) secondary to the laser treatment, and a test spot or patch may be performed on patients who are at high risk or those who are especially concerned about dyspigmentation [28]. The exact time to start fractional laser treatments is unknown. However, there is evidence that NAFL is well tolerated even in scars less than a year old, so long as the scars are epithelialized and not newly healing [9].

Relative contraindications to NAFL include the use of systemic isotretinoin within the last 6 months and use of systemic steroids due to increased risk of compromised wound healing [6, 29, 30]. Furthermore, patients who are prone to keloid formation or hypertrophic scarring are not ideal candidates. Patients seeking treatment of facial scars with a history of herpes simplex should be prescribed prophylactic antivirals such as oral acyclovir or valacyclovir 1 day prior to treatment and until reepithelialization occurs (typically 5 days posttreatment). Those with a history of facial staphylococcal infections may be prescribed antibiotic prophylaxis such as azithromycin [6].

For pain relief, topical agents such as lidocaine and prilocaine cream (EMLA) can be applied under occlusion 1 h prior to procedure. Cold air can also be used during the procedure to minimize discomfort. The application of cold packs immediately following the laser session can further ease any discomfort [6].

Treatment settings will depend on the characteristics of each individual burn scar. For the 1550-nm erbium:glass laser, energy levels up to 70 mJ per MTZ may be utilized with approximately 4–8 passes per session. The thulium laser energy settings are generally 10–20 mJ per MTZ with around 4–8 passes per session [12]. Treatments should be spaced 2–4 weeks apart. The total number of sessions needed can vary from as few as 3 to as many as 12 or more. Scar thickness, size, and treatment goals will impact session count. Noticeable results are usually appreciated after only a couple sessions [31]. Treatments with both laser wavelengths may be stacked in 1 day or used separately in different sessions. The depth and density can be decreased when treating areas with thinner cutaneous tissue including the neck [13].

Post-laser care may include the application of steroid cream such as triamcinolone 0.1% cream to treated areas twice daily for 3–4 days to help counteract post-procedural swelling. Additionally, strict sun avoidance pre- and post-procedure for at least 1–2 weeks before and after a NAFL treatment must be emphasized. Patient should be instructed to apply a liberal amount broad-spectrum sunscreen for at least 3 months [11, 31]. Patients should also strive to keep skin well moisturized. Bronzing of the treatment areas over the few days following treatment is expected and transient [32].

4 Clinical Examples

Case 1: A 30-year-old, Fitzpatrick phototype (FP) III woman was referred for treatment of extensive burn scars on the upper and lower extremities. Eight months prior, she had suffered second degree burn scars from a propane tank explosion at a picnic, and her burns were treated nonsurgically. She was managing the scars with silicone gel sheeting, scar massage, and compression garments. She had been prescribed oral gabapentin for burning and pruritus. The patient followed closely with a psychiatrist for her significant psychological distress following the traumatic accident. Physical exam showed hypertrophic, erythematous, and dyspigmented scars of the bilateral lower and upper extremities, including the dorsal hands and digits, affecting approximately 30% body surface area (BSA). The dark hyperpigmentation was especially severe on the lower extremities (Figs. 1a and 2a).

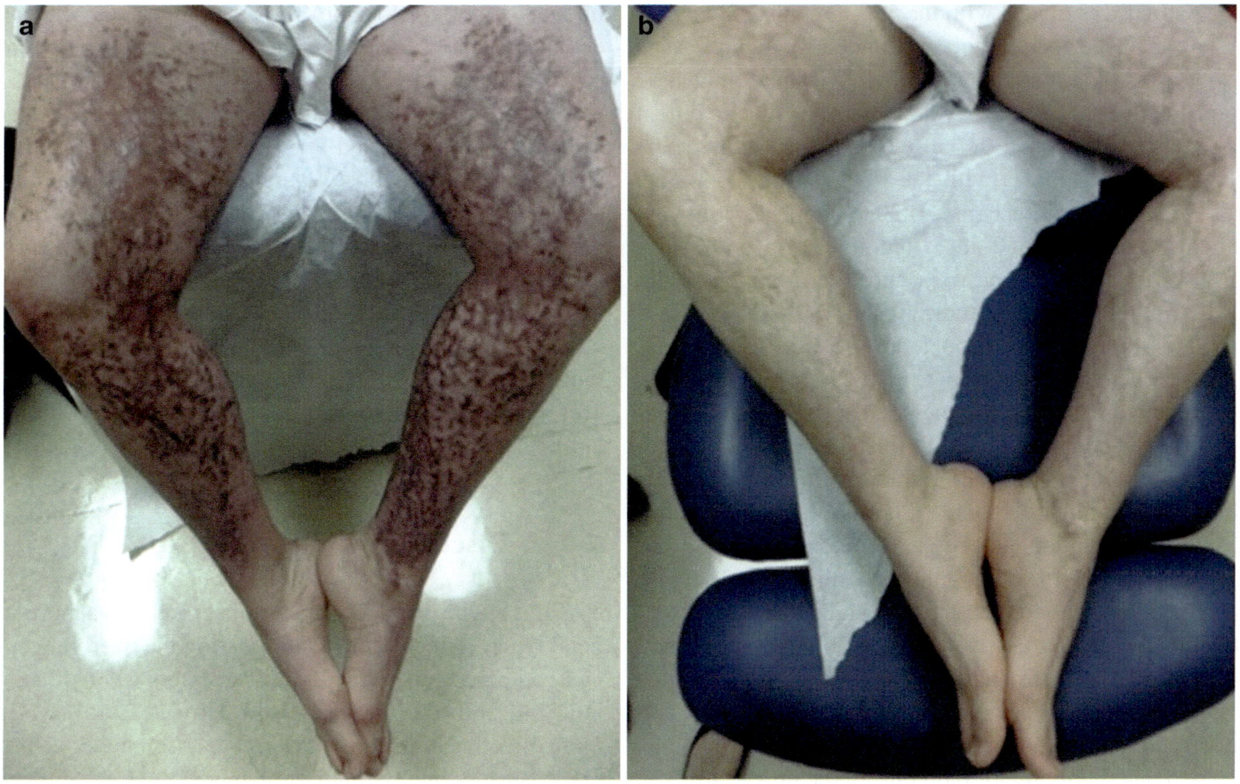

Fig. 1 (**a**) Burn scars on the bilateral lower extremities before treatment. (**b**) After 12 months

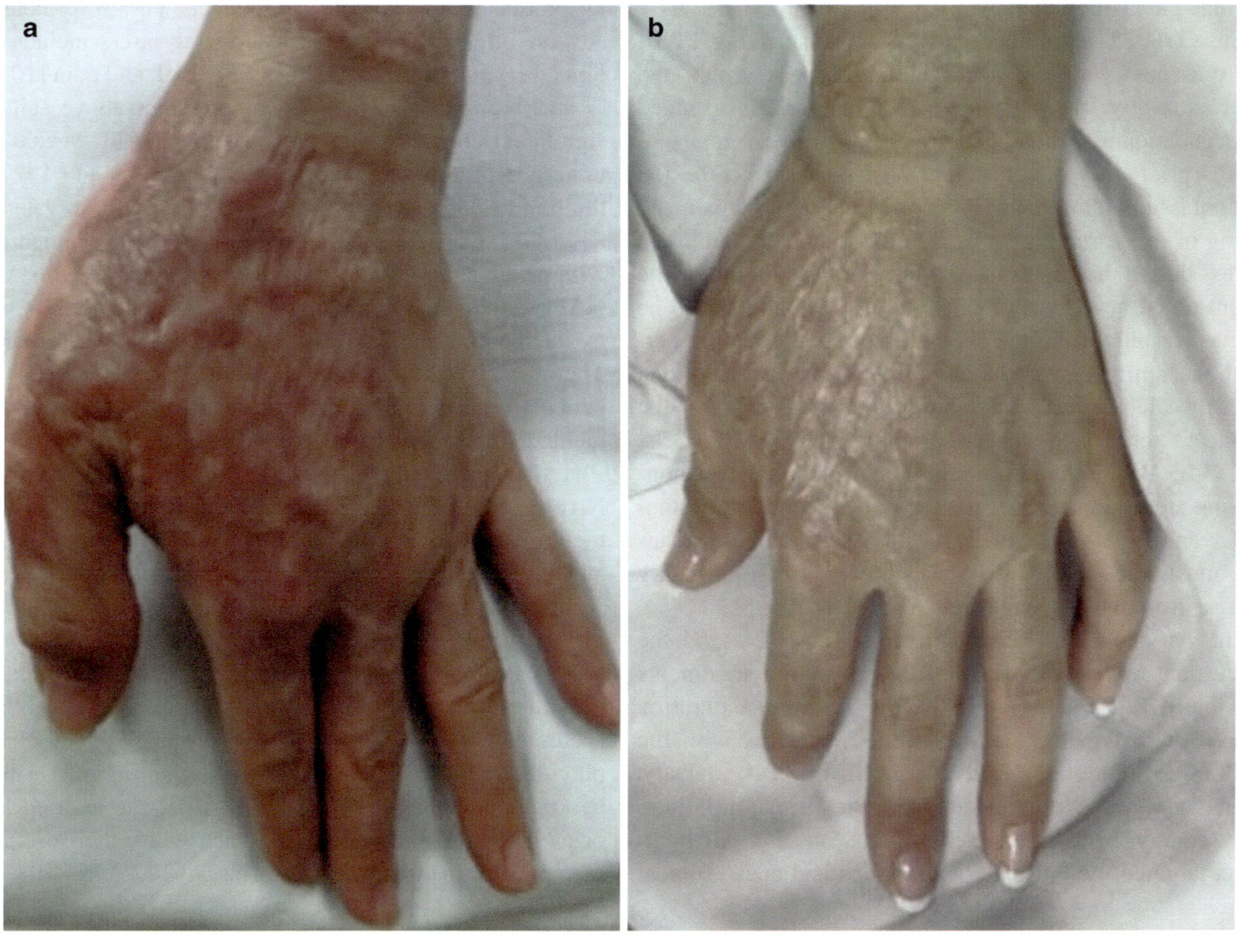

Fig. 2 (**a**) Burn scars on the dorsal hand before treatment. (**b**) After 12 months

The patient was treated with the 595-nm pulsed dye laser (PDL) (Vbeam Perfecta, Syneron Candela, Wayland, MA) and a NAFL dual wavelength device. Topical lidocaine 2.5%/prilocaine 2.5% cream was applied to the treatment areas under occlusion 1 h before each procedure. She received three treatments with the PDL (7 mm spot size, energy 8 J, pulse duration 6 ms, 30:20 dynamic cooling), six treatments with the 1550-nm erbium:glass laser (energy 30 mJ,14% density, 4–8 passes), and five treatments with the 1927-nm thulium laser (energy 10 mJ, 30% density, 4–8 passes) to the bilateral upper and lower extremities. Treatments were spaced approximately 1 month apart. Immediate posttreatment care included application of triamcinolone 0.1% cream twice daily for 3–4 days and broad-spectrum sunscreen. Adjuvant therapy included a one-time 1 mL of triamcinolone acetonide (20 mg/mL) injected intralesionally to a symptomatic hypertrophic scar on the left hand. Tacrolimus 0.1% ointment was applied twice daily to hyperpigmented scars on the legs throughout the course of treatment. Treated burn scars became softer, thinner, and more normal in texture and pigmentation with significant overall cosmetic improvement (Figs. 1b and 2b). The patient tolerated the laser treatments very well with no downtime. She experienced only minor pain during the procedure. The patient also reported improved mood and decreased pain and pruritus associated with her scars and was able to discontinue gabapentin therapy.

Case 2: A 33-year-old primarily Spanish-speaking, FP III man presented with burn scars on the left neck, trunk, and upper extremity. The patient, a sanitation worker, sustained an occupational, second-degree chemical burn injury 4 months prior after being accidentally splashed on the job with potassium phosphate. He reported intermittent pain and itching of the scarred areas as well as significant emotional distress due to the appearance of his scars. Additionally, the patient noted new areas of hair loss on the scalp, which he believed resulted from the chemical splash. He had no personal or family history of autoimmune disease. Physical exam revealed hypertrophic and erythematous scars of the left neck, torso, and upper extremity affecting 7% BSA (Fig. 3a). Well-defined, circular, non-inflammatory, non-scarring alopecic patches were also noted on the left postauricular and right vertex of the scalp. The alopecia patches were most consistent with alopecia areata, likely secondary to stress from the accident (Fig. 4a).

The patient was treated with a 595-nm PDL and the NAFL dual wavelength device. He received two treatments with the PDL (5 mm spot size, energy 7.5 J, pulse duration 6 ms, 30:20 dynamic cooling), four treatments with the 1550-nm erbium:glass laser (energy 30 mJ, 14% density, 4–8 passes), and two treatments with the 1927-nm thulium laser (energy 10 mJ, 30% density, 4–8 passes). All treatments targeted the left upper extremities and neck. Topical lidocaine 2.5%/prilocaine 2.5% cream was applied under occlusion to the treatment area 1 h prior to procedure. At two of his sessions, both non-ablative lasers (1550 and 1927 wavelengths) were used sequentially over the affected areas. Treatments were spaced approximately 1 month apart and were well tolerated. Posttreatment care included application of triamcinolone 0.1% cream twice daily for 3 days and sun protection with broad-spectrum sunscreen. Adjuvant therapy included continued scar massage. There was vast improvement in the appearance of the scars in regard to both texture and skin color (Fig. 3b). His alopecia areata resolved with four monthly sessions of intralesional triamcinolone acetonide injections (concentration 10 mg/mL, volume 0.5–2.5 mL) (Fig. 4b).

5 Discussion

NAFL is a type of fractional laser that produces a more superficial injury to the dermis while sparing the overlying epidermis compared to ablative fractional lasers (AFL) that cause injury to both the epidermis and dermis [7, 15]. AFLs are more effective at treating thicker, hypertrophic, or contracted scars because they stimulate a more vigorous remodeling response [5, 9]. However, NAFLs are associated with less post-procedural downtime and have a significantly lower risk of producing undesirable side effects [10, 33]. Potential adverse effects of fractional resurfacing lasers include prolonged erythema, swelling, blistering, PIH, and pain [10, 11].

The burn scars in the clinical examples above achieved significant clinical improvement with a NAFL device containing two lasers, the 1550-nm erbium:glass and 1927-nm thulium. This laser combination of two wavelengths addresses scar thickness, texture, and hyperpigmentation with a low side effect profile. When compared with AFLs, NAFLs are better at targeting dyschromia and are less likely to induce unwanted post-procedural pigmentary changes. Therefore, NAFLs may be especially advantageous in patients with skin of color who tend to develop more pigmented burn scars and are at an increased risk of developing PIH after resurfacing [10, 11, 34–37]. While treatment with NAFLs still carry a risk of unwanted post-procedural pigment changes, lower fluences, reduced treatment densities, and fewer treatment passes can minimize this risk [9, 10, 38].

In the example provided, burn scars were also treated with the 595-nm PDL device. Numerous studies have shown that PDLs can significantly reduce burn scar erythema, pain, pruritus, and thickness [39]. PDLs prevent excessive collagen accumulation and promote collagen remodeling via selective photothermolysis of scar vasculature resulting in scar tissue hypoxia and collagen fiber heating. PDL can be used alone or as part of a multimodal approach with other lasers and therapies for the treatment of burn scars [4, 5, 15, 40].

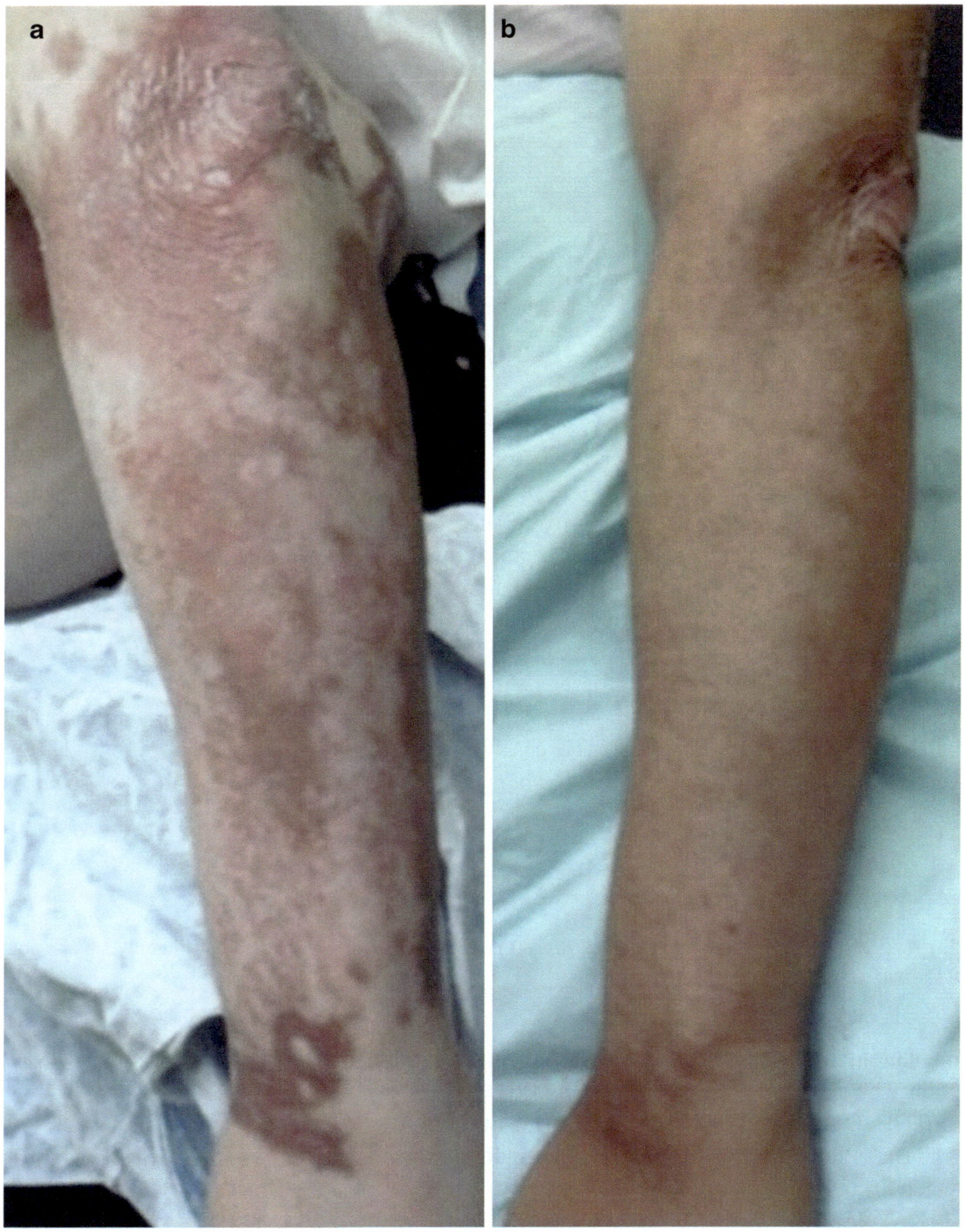

Fig. 3 (**a**) Burn scars on the left upper extremity before treatment. (**b**) After 6 months

In the first clinical example, tacrolimus ointment was used in conjunction with the laser treatments to address hyperpigmentation and reduce scarring in the bilateral lower extremities. Tacrolimus is a calcineurin inhibitor that prevents the activation of T-cells [41]. Its topical form is most commonly used to treat atopic dermatitis but has many off-label indications such as scarring due to its immunomodulating effects that may reduce inflammation and low side effect profile [42, 43]. There is limited evidence that suggests tacrolimus may ameliorate scarring by modulating collagen pathways and synthesis [44, 45]. However, the exact mechanism is not known, and further studies are needed to define its role in managing scars. There is one report of a keloid that resolved after application of topical tacrolimus, possibly due to its ability to inhibit *gli*-1 signal transduction, which is overexpressed in keloids [46]. A few studies have utilized topical tacrolimus to successfully treat pigmentation conditions including acquired facial hyperpigmentation and erythema dyschromicum perstans [20, 47].

Ultimately, the NAFL 1550-nm erbium:glass/1927-nm thulium device is effective and well-tolerated method for burn scar treatment. It is an excellent alternative to ablative fractional lasers offering the benefit of minimal downtime and decreased risk of dyschromia in darker skin types. The thulium laser specifically addresses hyperpig-

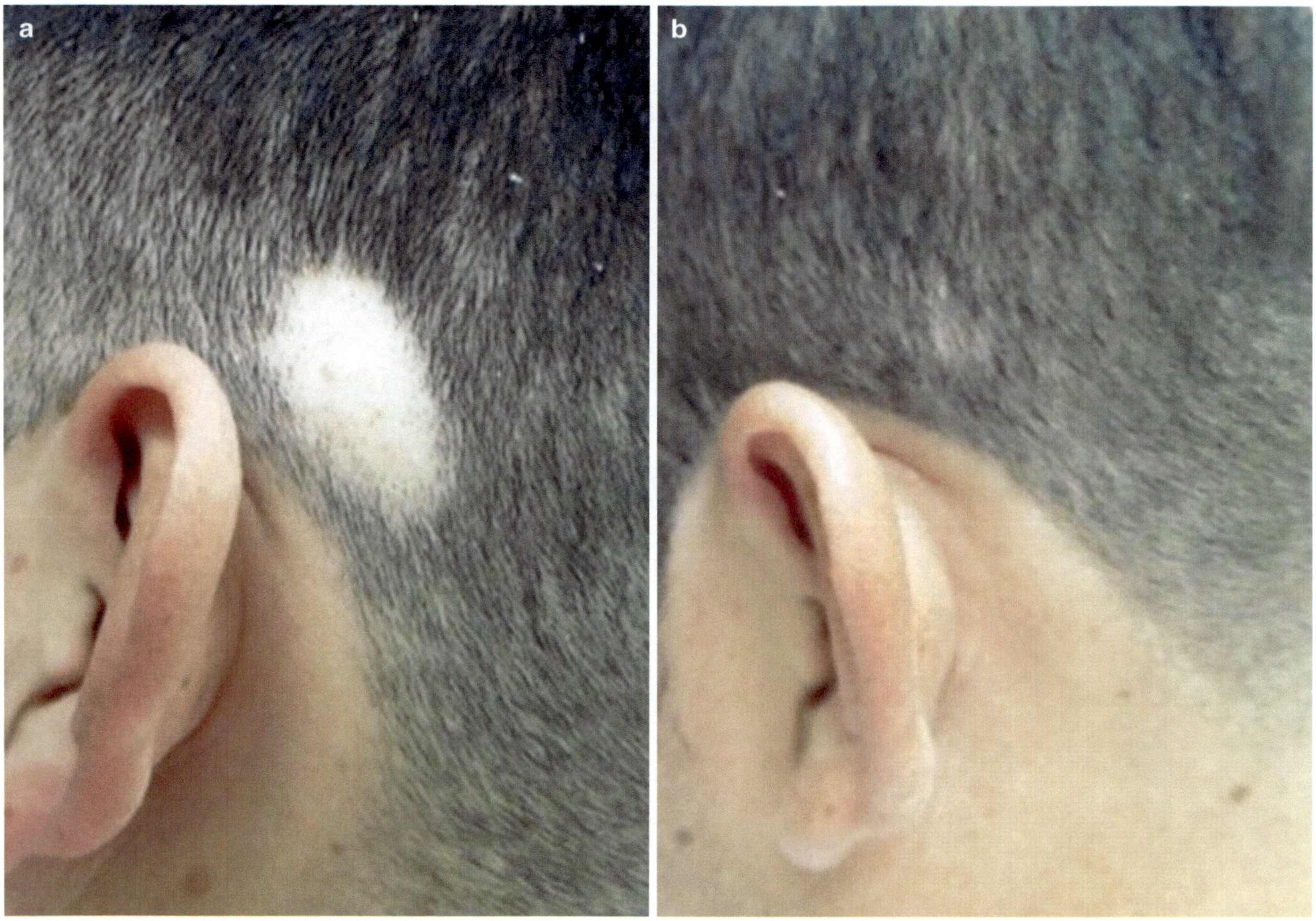

Fig. 4 (**a**) Non-scarring alopecic patch on the left postauricular scalp. (**b**) After four monthly sessions of intralesional triamcinolone acetonide injections

mentation, which is advantageous in patients with skin of color who are more prone to developing PIH.

THE JOURNAL IS AN OPEN ACCESS JOURNAL

THE PUBLISHING EDITOR IS: philippa.stevens@sagepub.co.uk

KAYVAN SHOKROLLAH IS EDITOR IN CHIEF OF THAT JOURNAL

References

1. Willows BM, Ilyas M, Sharma A. Laser in the management of burn scars. Burns. 2017;43(7):1379–89. https://doi.org/10.1016/j.burns.2017.07.001.
2. Van Loey NE, Van Son MJ. Psychopathology and psychological problems in patients with burn scars: epidemiology and management. Am J Clin Dermatol. 2003;4(4):245–72. https://doi.org/10.2165/00128071-200304040-00004.
3. Esselman PC, Thrombs BD, Magyar-Russell G, et al. Burn rehabilitation: state of the science. Am J Phys Med Rehabil. 2006;85(4):383–413. https://doi.org/10.1097/01.phm.0000202095.51037.a3.
4. Brewin MP, Lister TS. Prevention or treatment of hypertrophic burn scarring: a review of when and how to treat with the pulsed dye laser. Burns. 2014;40(5):797–804. https://doi.org/10.1016/j.burns.2013.12.017.
5. Issler-Fisher AC, Waibel JS, Donelan MB, et al. Laser modulation of hypertrophic scars technique and practice. Clin Plast Surg. 2017;44(4):757–66. https://doi.org/10.1016/j.cps.2017.05.007.
6. Alexiades-Armenakas MR, Dover JS, Arndt KA, et al. The spectrum of laser skin resurfacing: nonablative, fractional, and ablative laser resurfacing. J Am Acad Dermatol. 2008;58(5):719–37; quiz 738–40. https://doi.org/10.1016/j.jaad.2008.01.003.
7. Manstein D, Herron GS, Sink RK, et al. Fractional photothermolysis: a new concept for cutaneous remodeling using microscopic patterns of thermal injury. Lasers Surg Med. 2004;34(5):426–38. https://doi.org/10.1002/lsm.20048.
8. Taudorf EH, Danielsen PL, Paulsen IF, et al. Non-ablative fractional laser provides long-term improvement of mature burn scars–a randomized controlled trial with histological assessment. Lasers Surg Med. 2015;47(2):141–7. https://doi.org/10.1002/lsm.22289.
9. Anderson RR, Donelan MB, Hivnor C, et al. Laser treatment of traumatic scars with an emphasis on ablative fractional laser resurfacing: consensus report. JAMA Dermatol. 2014;150(2):187–93. https://doi.org/10.1001/jamadermatol.2013.7761.
10. Bogdan Allemann I, Kaufman J. Fractional photothermolysis—an update. Lasers Med Sci. 2010;25(1):137–44. https://doi.org/10.1007/s10103-009-0734-8.
11. Alam M, Warycha M. Complications of lasers and light treatments. Dermatol Ther. 2011;24(6):571–80. https://doi.org/10.1111/j.1529-8019.2012.01476.x.
12. Preissig J, Hamilton K, Markus R. Current laser resurfacing technologies: a review that delves beneath the surface.

Semin Plast Surg. 2012;26(3):109–16. https://doi.org/10.1055/s-0032-1329413.
13. Waibel J, Wulkan AJ, Lupo M, et al. Treatment of burn scars with the 1,550 nm nonablative fractional erbium laser. Lasers Surg Med. 2012;44(6):441–6. https://doi.org/10.1002/lsm.22038.
14. Finney R, Torbeck R, Saedi N. Non-ablative fractional resurfacing in the treatment of scar contracture. Lasers Surg Med. 2016;48(2):170–3. https://doi.org/10.1002/lsm.22400.
15. Stewart N, Lim AC, Lowe PM, et al. Lasers and laser-like devices: part one. Australas J Dermatol. 2013;54(3):173–83. https://doi.org/10.1111/ajd.12034.
16. Polder KD, Bruce S. Treatment of melasma using a novel 1,927-nm fractional thulium fiber laser: a pilot study. Dermatol Surg. 2012;38(2):199–206. https://doi.org/10.1111/j.1524-4725.2011.02178.x.
17. Lee HM, Haw S, Kim JK, et al. Split-face study using a 1,927-nm thulium fiber fractional laser to treat photoaging and melasma in Asian skin. Dermatol Surg. 2013;39(6):879–88. https://doi.org/10.1111/dsu.12176.
18. Ho SG, Yeung CK, Chan NP, et al. A retrospective study of the management of Chinese melasma patients using a 1927 nm fractional thulium fiber laser. J Cosmet Laser Ther. 2013;15(4):200–6. https://doi.org/10.3109/14764172.2012.761346.
19. Niwa Massaki AB, Eimputh S, Fabi SG, et al. Treatment of melasma with the 1,927-nm fractional thulium fiber laser: a retrospective analysis of 20 cases with long-term follow-up. Lasers Surg Med. 2013;45(2):95–101. https://doi.org/10.1002/lsm.22100.
20. Lee YJ, Park JH, Lee D, et al. Acquired bilateral dyspigmentation on face and neck: clinically appropriate approaches. J Korean Med Sci. 2016;31(12):2042–50. https://doi.org/10.3346/jkms.2016.31.12.2042.
21. Lee SJ, Chung WS, Lee JD, et al. A patient with cupping-related post-inflammatory hyperpigmentation successfully treated with a 1,927 nm thulium fiber fractional laser. J Cosmet Laser Ther. 2014;16(2):66–8. https://doi.org/10.3109/14764172.2013.854121.
22. Brauer JA, McDaniel DH, Blood BS. Nonablative 1927 nm fractional resurfacing for the treatment of facial photopigmentation. J Drugs Dermatol. 2014;13(11):1317–22.
23. Boen M, Wilson MJV, Goldman MP, et al. Rejuvenation of the male scalp using 1,927 nm non-ablative fractional thulium fiber laser. Lasers Surg Med. 2017;49(5):475–9. https://doi.org/10.1002/lsm.22624.
24. Wu DC, Friedmann DP, Fabi SG, et al. Comparison of intense pulsed light with 1,927-nm fractionated thulium fiber laser for the rejuvenation of the chest. Dermatol Surg. 2014;40(2):129–33. https://doi.org/10.1111/dsu.12398.
25. Polder KD, Harrison A, Eubanks LE, et al. 1,927-nm fractional thulium fiber laser for the treatment of nonfacial photodamage: a pilot study. Dermatol Surg. 2011;37(3):342–8. https://doi.org/10.1111/j.1524-4725.2011.01884.x.
26. Narurkar VA, Alster TS, Bernstein EF, et al. Safety and efficacy of a 1550nm/1927nm dual wavelength laser for the treatment of photodamaged skin. J Drugs Dermatol. 2018;17(1):41–6.
27. Tao J, Champlain A, Weddington C, et al. Treatment of burn scars in Fitzpatrick phototype III patients with a combination of pulsed dye laser and non-ablative fractional resurfacing 1550 nm erbium:glass/1927 nm thulium laser devices. Scars Burns Heal. 2018;4:1–6. https://doi.org/10.1177/2059513118758510.
28. Shokrollahi K. The laser test patch: principles and philosophy to maximise efficacy and reduce complications and scarring from laser treatments. Ann Plast Surg. 2016;77(4):373–5. https://doi.org/10.1097/SAP.0000000000000894.
29. Rubenstein R, Roenigk HH Jr, Stegman SJ, et al. Atypical keloids after dermabrasion of patients taking isotretinoin. J Am Acad Dermatol. 1986;15(2 pt 1):280–5. https://doi.org/10.1016/S0190-9622(86)70167-9.
30. Valeant Pharmaceuticals International. Important safety information. http://www.fraxel.com/fraxelphysician/indications-results/important-safety-information. Accessed 16 March 2018
31. Valeant Pharmaceuticals International. Frequently asked questions. http://www.fraxel.com/find-a-doctor/faq/3. Accessed 30 March 2018
32. Tanzi EL, Wanitphakdeedecha R, Alster TS. Fraxel laser indications and long-term follow-up. Aesthet Surg J. 2008;28(6):675–8. https://doi.org/10.1016/j.asj.2008.09.006.
33. Shin JU, Gantsetseg D, Jung JY, et al. Comparison of non-ablative and ablative fractional laser treatments in a postoperative scar study. Lasers Surg Med. 2014;46(10):741–9. https://doi.org/10.1002/lsm.22297.
34. Kaushik SB, Alexis AF. Nonablative fractional laser resurfacing in skin of color: evidence-based review. J Clin Aesthet Dermatol. 2017;10(6):51–67.
35. Alexis AF, Coley MK, Nijhawan RI, et al. Nonablative fractional laser resurfacing for acne scarring in patients with Fitzpatrick skin Phototypes IV-VI. Dermatol Surg. 2016;42(3):392–402. https://doi.org/10.1097/DSS.0000000000000640.
36. Alajlan AM, Alsuwaidan SN. Acne scars in ethnic skin treated with both non-ablative fractional 1,550 nm and ablative fractional CO2 lasers: comparative retrospective analysis with recommended guidelines. Lasers Surg Med. 2011;43(8):787–91. https://doi.org/10.1002/lsm.21092.
37. Davis EC, Callender VD. Postinflammatory hyperpigmentation: a review of the epidemiology, clinical features, and treatment options in skin of color. J Clin Aesthet Dermatol. 2010;3(7):20–31.
38. Bach DQ, Garcia MS, Eisen DB. Hyperpigmented burn scar improved with a fractionated 1550 nm non-ablative laser. Dermatol Online J. 2012;18(7):12.
39. Parrett BM, Donelan MB. Pulsed dye laser in burn scars: current concepts and future directions. Burns. 2010;36(4):443–9. https://doi.org/10.1016/j.burns.2009.08.015.
40. Miletta NR, Donelan MB, Hivnor CM. Management of trauma and burn scars: the dermatologist's role in expanding patient access to care. Cutis. 2017;100(1):18–20.
41. Berman B, Viera MH, Amini S, et al. Prevention and management of hypertrophic scars and keloids after burns in children. J Craniofac Surg. 2008;19(4):989–1006. https://doi.org/10.1097/SCS.0b013e318175f3a7.
42. Carroll CL, Fleischer AB Jr. Tacrolimus ointment: the treatment of atopic dermatitis and other inflammatory cutaneous disease. Expert Opin Pharmacother. 2004;5(10):2127–31. https://doi.org/10.1517/14656566.5.10.2127.
43. Viera MH, Amini S, Valins W, et al. Innovative therapies in the treatment of keloids and hypertrophic scars. J Clin Aesthet Dermatol. 2010;3(5):20–6.
44. Wong VW, You F, Januszyk M, et al. Tacrolimus fails to regulate collagen expression in dermal fibroblasts. J Surg Res. 2013;184(1):678–90. https://doi.org/10.1016/j.jss.2013.04.006.
45. Gisquet H, Liu H, Blondel WC, et al. Intradermal tacrolimus prevent scar hypertrophy in a rabbit ear model: a clinical, histological and spectroscopical analysis. Skin Res Technol. 2011;17(2):160–6. https://doi.org/10.1111/j.1600-0846.2010.00479.x.
46. Kim A, DiCarlo J, Cohen C, et al. Are keloids really "gli-loids"?: High-level expression of gli-1 oncogene in keloids. J Am Acad Dermatol. 2001;45(5):707–11. https://doi.org/10.1067/mjd.2001.117736.
47. Mahajan VK, Chauhan PS, Mehta KS, et al. Erythema dyschromicum perstans: response to topical tacrolimus. Indian J Dermatol. 2015;60(5):525. https://doi.org/10.4103/0019-5154.164452.

Laser Depilation in Scar and Burn Management: Scar Folliculitis, Heterotopic Hair Growth, and Keloids

Corina Lavelle, Umarah Muhammad,
Yvonne Stubbington, and Kayvan Shokrollahi

1 Heterotopic Hair Growth

Heterotopic hair growth is characterised by excessive hair growth in an abnormal anatomical location. The most common causes in the general population include an overproduction or increased sensitivity to circulating androgens, although most patterns of hair growth vary depending on sex and ethnicity [1]. In patients who have required reconstructive surgery, this can lead to hair-bearing donor tissue being present in non-hear-bearing areas, or an excess. Examples include: ear reconstruction with hair-bearing scalp skin leading to hairy ears; skin grafts such as full-thickness skin from the groin causing course or even pubic hair on the reconstructed areas including the face; and internal reconstructions such as tongue, floor of mouth, nose, lumen of the penis or neovagina after reconstruction growing hair.

1.1 Pseudo-Folliculitis and Scar Folliculitis

Pseudo-folliculitis is an inflammatory skin condition characterised by follicular and perifollicular papules and pustules. The lesions may be erythematous, skin-coloured, or hyperpigmented, and may be associated with pain and pruritis [2]. It is commonly associated with shaving and frequently affects the beard region. The common pathogenesis of pseudo-folliculitis is thought to involve trans- and extra-follicular penetration, whereby hair re-entry causes irritation of the epidermal layer and leads to formation of intra-epidermal micro-abscesses [2, 3]. The hair follicles of individuals with tightly curled hair are curved, making trans- and extra-follicular penetration more likely. Pseudo-folliculitis is therefore seen most commonly in men of African origin; however, it can affect both men and women of any ethnic group [4]. In chronic or severe cases, the inflammatory response can progress to hypertrophic scaring or keloid formation [2, 3]. Scarring in areas of hair-bearing tissue is a significant problem that causes and contributes to folliculitis and has a major impact on the quality of life of patients who suffer from it. In some patients who also suffer from keloid scarring, it can be devastating through the continuous stimulus for more scarring and keloids and the hinderance of otherwise successful treatments for keloids in areas where hair remains. Scar folliculitis is therefore a distinct clinical entity.

Folliculitis is therefore relevant in the following ways that can be helped with lasers:

- As a cause of scarring: keloid scarring of the face.
- As a result of scarring: scar folliculitis with disordered and buried hair growth.

The cosmetic appearance and other sequelae of both heterotopic hair growth and pseudo-folliculitis can cause significant distress to patients, who are often in search for a definitive method of treatment. Where an underlying medical condition, for example polycystic ovarian syndrome (PCOS) can be identified, management of the primary problem often takes precedence [1]. Pseudo-folliculitis most commonly occurs as a result of attempts at hair removal, and therefore patients are advised to avoid shaving, waxing, or tweezing. Adapting the shaving technique may also alleviate symptoms in some individuals [5]. However, conventional strategies—such as those advised by the British Association of Dermatology Guidelines (depilatory creams, medications such as steroid preparations and antiseptic lotions to reduce

C. Lavelle
The Christie NHS Foundation Trust, Manchester, UK
e-mail: CORINALAVELLE@DOCTORS.ORG.UK

U. Muhammad · Y. Stubbington
Mersey Regional Centre for Burns and Plastic Surgery, Whiston Hospital, Liverpool, UK
e-mail: yvonne.stubbington@sthk.nhs.uk

K. Shokrollahi (✉)
Burns and Plastic Surgery Unit, Whiston Hospital, Liverpool, UK

K. Shokrollahi (ed.), *Laser Management of Scars*, https://doi.org/10.1007/978-3-030-52919-2_15

inflammation, short courses of oral antibiotics where infection is present, and occasionally retinoid creams or retinoid and antibiotic combinations) [5] are typically not relevant or appropriate for patients with scar folliculitis.

Laser therapy is increasingly seen as the gold standard in the management of excessive hair growth. The aim of laser hair removal is to use specific wavelengths of light to destroy hair follicles and prevent future hair growth by causing irreversible damage to follicular stem cells [6]. The optimal wavelength of light is well absorbed by melanin found in hair follicles but does not interact with other chromophores in the skin such as haemoglobin and water. The pulse duration required is sufficient to destroy the hair follicle without damaging surrounding tissues, and this can be achieved by choosing a pulse duration shorter than the cooling time of the hair follicle [6]. Laser therapy has been shown to be effective in the management of both heterotopic hair growth and pseudo-folliculitis; however, several important factors must be taken into consideration.

1.2 Which Laser?

The first consideration is the type of laser source used. The first laser described for the use of destruction of hair follicles was a long-pulsed ruby laser (694 nm) and provided promising results [7]. Since this time, a number of new laser systems with varying wavelengths have been developed. A systematic review of clinical trials related to hair removal lasers between 1998 and 2003 synthesised trial results based on the type of laser used [8]. The results showed that hair reduction at least 6 months following treatment were 57.5%, 42.3%, 54.7%, and 52.8% after three sessions for diode (800–810 nm), neodymium-doped yttrium aluminum garnet (Nd:YAG; 1064 nm), pulsed alexandrite (755 nm), and ruby lasers, respectively. The diode laser appeared to be the most effective in this review with the Nd:YAG demonstrating the least promise. A randomised control trial (RCT) compared the efficacy and side effect profile of long-pulsed diode and long-pulse alexandrite lasers [9]. Twenty women underwent treatment with the alexandrite and diode lasers by randomly assigning axillary areas to both laser types. Success rates were measured using hair counts and skin punch biopsies. Results showed an equivalent and significant reduction in hair growth with the use of both lasers.

A number of studies have supported the use of lasers for the treatment of pseudo-folliculitis [6, 10–14]. The use of long-pulsed Nd:YAG has frequently been described for the management of pseudo-folliculitis within the world literature [12, 13]. In dark skin, epidermal melanin acts as a competing chromophore making the risk of epidermal injury in the form of dyspigmentation and scarring more likely [13]. In those with higher Fitzpatrick skin phototypes, longer wavelength lasers such as the Nd:YAG lasers are often considered safer and thus more suitable [13, 14],. Other laser systems have also been described. An RCT compared the use of alexandrite and intense pulsed light (IPL) by randomly assigning one of the therapies to either half of the face in 15 male patients [15]. A statistically significant decrease in the number of papules was observed using both lasers; however, alexandrite required fewer treatment sessions to achieve greater clinical efficacy with fewer rates of recurrence. Although the IPL system demonstrated less clinical efficacy compared to the alexandrite laser in this study, its role within laser hair removal is yet to be determined, with its benefits including a smaller start-up cost and the ability to treat a variety of other conditions by changing the filter used [15, 16].

The number and timing of laser treatments play important roles in determining the efficacy of a given system in laser hair removal. A retrospective study divided 23 patients into four groups according to the number of laser treatments that they had received and used digital photography and hair counting to compare results [17]. A positive correlation was observed between the number of treatments and degree of hair reduction; however, most side effects could be seen in cases of six or more treatments. The authors of this study suggest that five is the optimal number of treatments in order to achieve successful hair removal whilst minimising adverse effects such as blistering and hyper- or hyper-pigmentation. Another study also used hair counting to assess the mean hair reduction of 24 patients at 45-, 60-, and 90-day intervals and showed results of 78.1%, 45.8%, and 28.7%, respectively [18]. Whilst these results suggest that smaller treatment intervals provide greater hair reduction, a general consensus on the ideal treatment interval is yet to be established.

Whilst the aim of laser hair removal is to target follicular melanin, melanocytes and keratinocytes within the epidermis may also absorb laser radiation leading to unwanted side effects, for example blistering or changes to skin pigmentation [6, 19]. A study looked at the side effect profiles of Q-switched Nd:YAG, long-pulsed ruby, and alexandrite lasers in a large patient population [20]. Treatment pain was commonly experienced during laser therapy; however, this is usually mild. Other common side effects in all laser groups included oedema and erythema, but these often clear within 1–4 h of treatment and are expected sequelae to the use of laser photo-thermolysis. Adverse effects such as blistering and skin discolouration occur more frequently in dark skin phototypes [19, 20], and differences in incidence based on seasonal variation and anatomical location might also suggest a link to sun exposure. Few studies have reported long-term side effects following laser therapy; however, rare complications including paradoxical hypertrichosis have been documented in the literature [21]. We do not feel Q-switched lasers have a significant role to play in depilation. Most conventional lasers marketed for hair removal in particular as alexandrite and diode lasers will be suitable for depilation in scar tissue. In general, long-pulsed Nd:YAG lasers are best used for the darkest of skin types (4–6) and alexandrite and diode lasers always used in preference due to their greater efficacy.

2 Keloid Scars

Keloid scars are a form of pathological scarring that occur as a result of altered wound healing following injury and grow in a pattern no dissimilar to benign tumours. The pathophysiology of these scar types is complex and involves the deposition of excessive amounts of collagen, although the exact cause remains elusive understood [22].

Keloid scars are seen to extend beyond the boundaries of the original wound and have a tendency to continue to develop without a regressive phase [22, 23]. Associated symptoms can include pruritus, pain, and restriction of movement. A number of factors are thought to contribute to the development of keloid scars, including skin injuries such as piercings, burns, surgery, insect bites, and inflammatory skin conditions such as acne [23]. Wound tension has also been linked to their development. Keloid scars have a higher incidence in patients with darker skin types and develop most commonly in patients between 10 and 30 years of age [23]. The presence of keloids can have a significant impact on the psychological well-being and self-esteem of patients [22].

Prophylaxis of pathological scarring is of upmost importance and is therefore more effective than treatment of subsequent scarring. Rapid primary closure of cutaneous defects in a way to avoid wound tension, debridement of contaminated wounds, and careful selection of suture material are all important in reducing the likelihood of pathological scarring [22, 23]. In individuals who are known to have a predisposition to keloid scarring, non-essential surgical procedures should be avoided and the risk of scarring explained, particularly in cosmetic procedures [22, 23]. Treatment options outlined by the British Association of Dermatologists include intralesional steroid and/or 5-fluorouracil injections, silicone dressings or gel, compression bandages and devices, radiotherapy, cryotherapy, laser therapy, and experimental treatments including bleomycin [24].

Intralesional steroid injection with triamcinolone, a potent anti-inflammatory, is a popular and effective treatment option for the management of keloid scars and is thought to work by preventing collagen synthesis and proliferation of fibroblasts [25]. Response rates following treatment are variable, and recurrence rates of between 9 and 50% have been documented in the literature [22]. Furthermore, the use of steroid injections in older scars that are less metabolically active is often less beneficial [26]. The management of keloid scaring therefore remains a challenge to clinicians and uncertainty remains with regard to which treatment is the most effective [27]. A meta-analysis in 2006 involved a PubMed search with the aim of reviewing the effectiveness of various treatments for keloids and hypertrophic scars [27]. Individual studies were graded based on their level of evidence, and results were delineated into those which were considered favourable and non-favourable. The meta-analysis of 70 treatment series found that there was a 70% chance of improvement of hypertrophic and keloid scarring with all treatment modalities. Despite this, no statistically significant difference was found to exist between the various treatments described.

Despite a relative paucity of evidence to support the use of laser therapy as a gold standard, it is increasingly recognised as one of the important treatment options for keloid scarring. A number of different laser systems have been studied for the treatment of keloid scars including both ablative and non-ablative lasers—CO_2, Er:YAG and pulsed dye laser (PDL), and Nd:YAG amongst others [28]. Concomitant ancillary background treatment remains important, especially intralesional therapy.

Patients with severe facial scar folliculitis will benefit from aggressive regular laser depilation. Even more important is the aggressive and pre-emptive treatment of patients who suffer from facial keloid scars. We would advise any patient with impending or new areas of folliculitis of the face, and who already have keloid scars should undertake regular and total facial depilation as prophylaxis against almost inevitable progression to new and extensive keloids elsewhere on the face. For these patients, there is a clock ticking: once their hair becomes grey or white, they will no longer be suitable for laser treatment.

For these patients at risk of keloid scarring, laser safety becomes even more important to minimise complications and risk of scarring. The definitive principles of laser test patching have been published elsewhere [29].

2.1 Clinical Examples

1. Facial Acid Attack/Scar Folliculitis (Fig. 1a, b)—Depilation with Alexandrite Laser
2. Heterotopic hair grown (Fig. 2)
3. Keloid Scar/Folliculitis Patient (Fig. 3)
4. Keloid scar folliculitis (Fig. 4)
5. Keloid scar folliculitis (Fig. 5)
6. Heterotopic hair growth (Fig. 6a–c)
7. Scar folliculitis (Fig. 7)

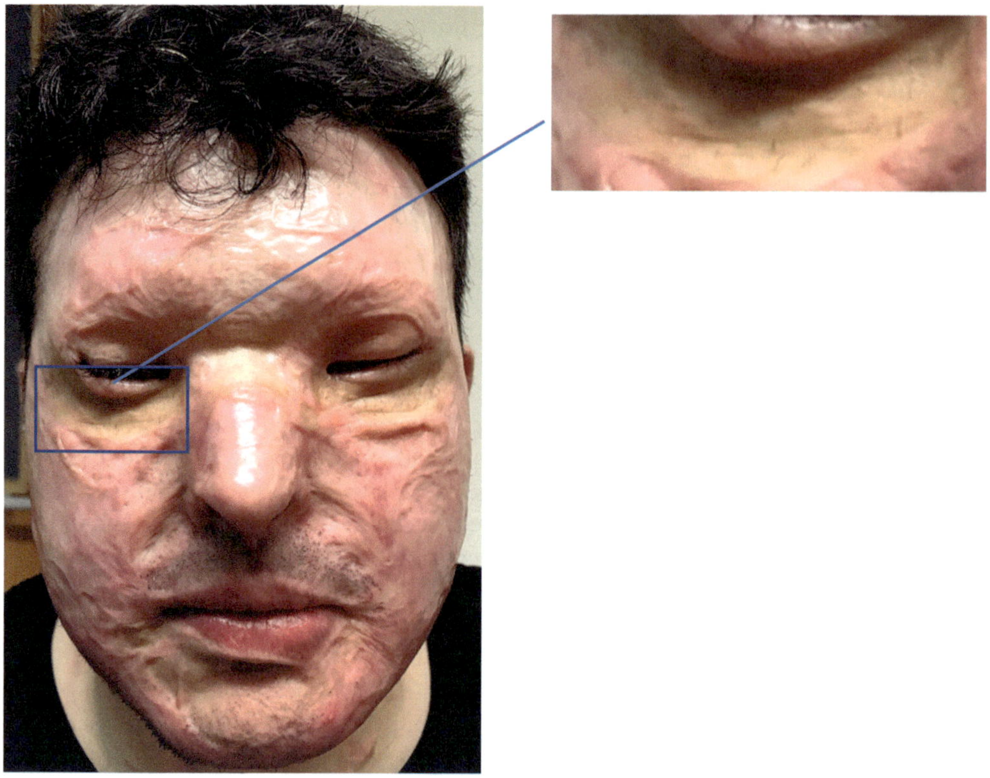

Fig. 1 (**a**, **b**) This patient has survived an acid attack and has found significant improvement of scar folliculitis from treatment of the beard area with alexandrite laser depilation. He also has ectopic hair from full-thickness skin grafts of the lower eyelids amenable to treatment. (Patients treated by the Professor Kayvan Shokrollahi and use is with permission from St Helens & Knowsley NHS Trust)

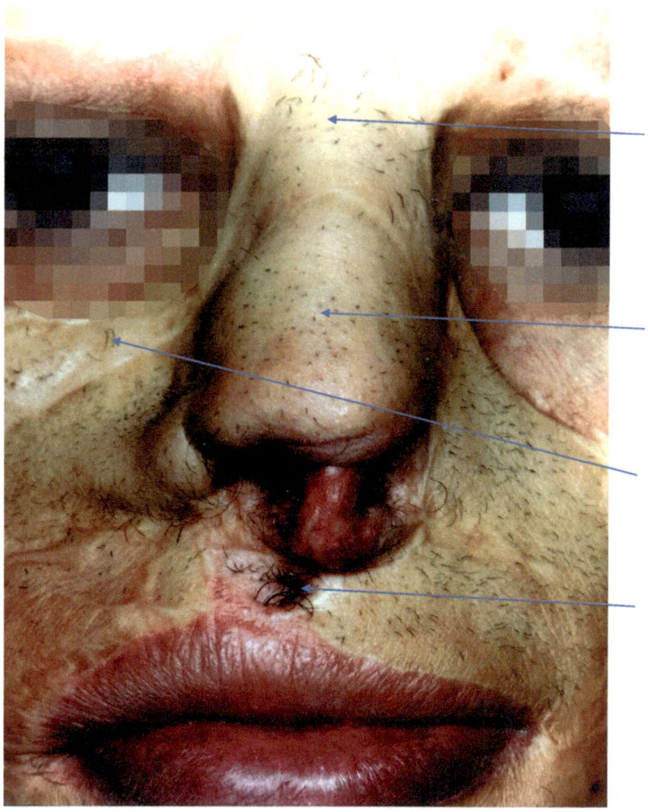

Fig. 2 This patient who has survived 80% burns was referred from another burns centre presenting with significant heterotopic hair growth with some additional folliculitis that is being successfully controlled by regular alexandrite laser depilation. (Patients treated by the Professor Kayvan Shokrollahi and use is with permission from St Helens & Knowsley NHS Trust)

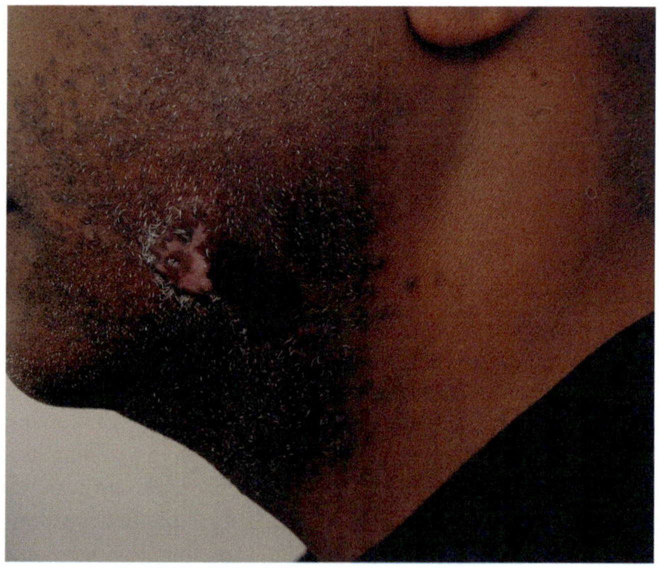

Fig. 3 Keloid scar folliculitis—white hair will not be responsive to laser therapy. Prophylactic or early depilationx is recommended for all patients whom might benefit early as possible before grey or white hairs replace the dark hairs. White or grey hair on the background of dark skin is a contraindication for laser depilation. (Patients treated by the Professor Kayvan Shokrollahi and use is with permission from St Helens & Knowsley NHS Trust)

3 Summary

The use of lasers for excessive or heterotopic hair growth, folliculitis, and pseudo-folliculitis has a long track record and is an important treatment modality for scar folliculitis

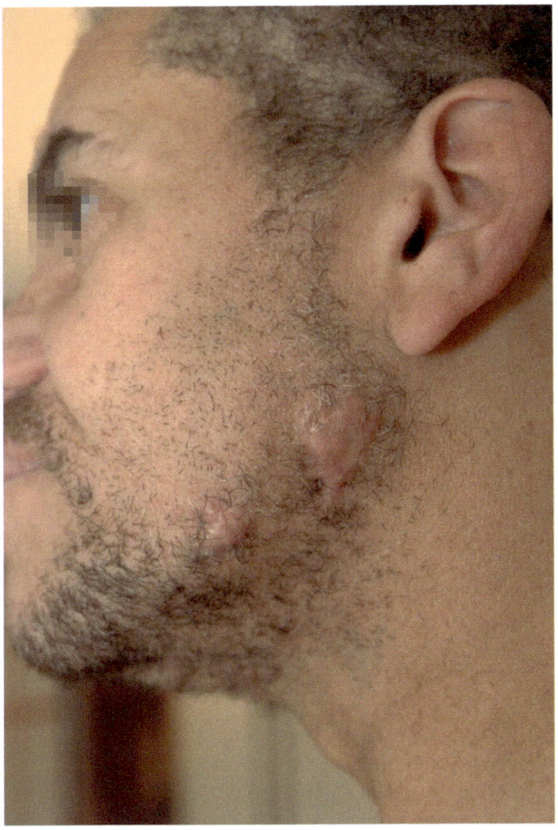

Fig. 4 Keloid scar folliculitis with mixed black and grey hair. (Patient treated by the Professor Kayvan Shokrollahi and use is with permission from St Helens & Knowsley NHS Trust)

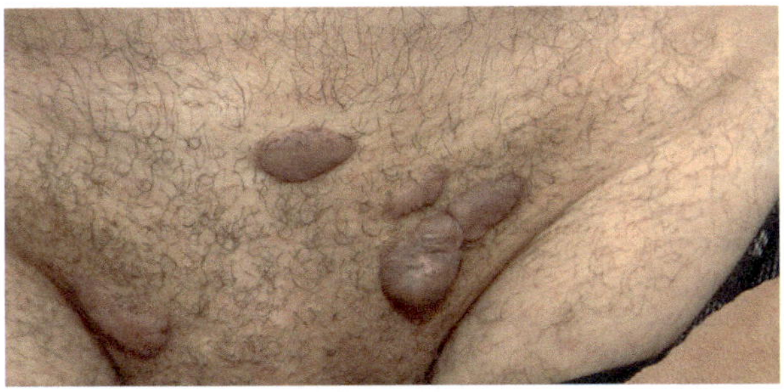

Fig. 5 Keloid scar folliculitis of the suprapubic area. Regular laser depilation is of considerable benefit regardless of the therapeutic strategy for the keloid scars. (Patients treated by the Professor Kayvan Shokrollahi and use is with permission from St Helens & Knowsley NHS Trust)

and ectopic hair growth in patients with scars or whom have received reconstructive surgery. The laser of choice will depend on factors such as skin type, anatomy, scar thickness, hair colour, and depth of the hairs—Nd:YAG is considered safer in the treatment of dark skin whilst alexandrite and diode lasers have proven to be most effective for hair removal in clinical trials.

Treatment of keloid scars can be challenging, and whilst intralesional therapies have played an important role in the management of keloids to date, improvement in scaring is not always guaranteed and also leads to skin changes such as telangiectasia which can themselves be amenable to laser treatment. Cost-effectiveness analyses will be of great benefit in future in a number of areas. For example, preventing one keloid scar by treating folliculitis that causes them is likely to save on decades worth of ongoing treatments.

Patients who have heterotopic hair growth as a result of reconstructive surgery may require prolonged courses of treatment in the absence of other effective strategies to deal with this problem. As always, prevention is better than cure, and all reconstructive strategies should be mindful of the problems caused by hair in an atypical location or in an excessive quantity.

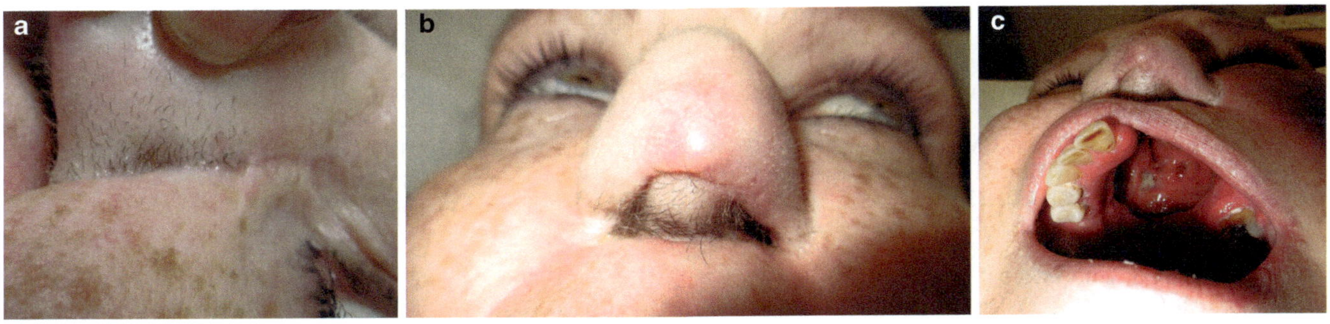

Fig. 6 (a) Nasal reconstruction with heterotopic hair from forehead flap. (b) Nasal reconstruction with heterotopic hair from forehead flap. (c) Nasopharyngeal hair from forehead flap reconstruction (obturator/prosthesis removed). (Patients treated by the Professor Kayvan Shokrollahi and use is with permission from St Helens & Knowsley NHS Trust)

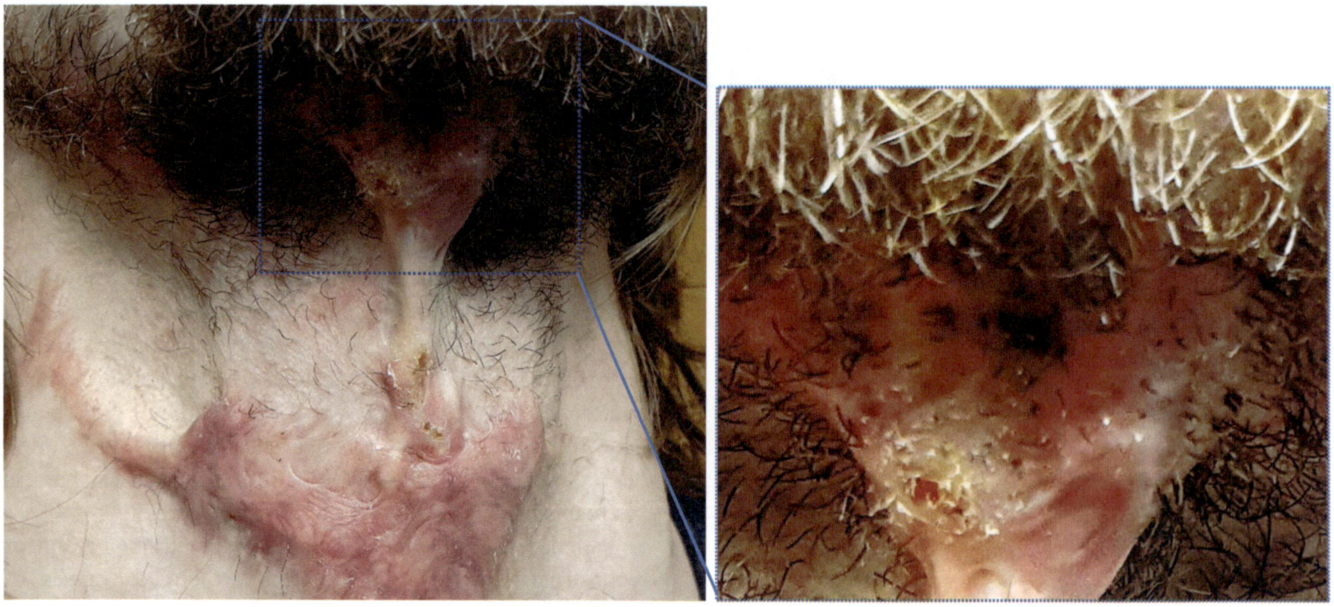

Fig. 7 Scar folliculitis in the beard and neck area from hypertrophic burns scars, worse under the chin, prior to a course of laser depilation. Patients treated by the Professor Kayvan Shokrollahi and use is with permission from St Helens & Knowsley NHS Trust

References

1. Shenenberger DW, Utecht LM. Removal of unwanted facial hair. Am Fam Physician. 2002;66:1907–11.
2. Alexis AF. Folliculitis keloidalis nuchae and pseudofolliculitis barbae- are prevention and effective treatment within reach? Dermatol Clin. 2014;32:183–91.
3. Bridgeman-Shah S. The medical and surgical therapy of pseudofolliculitis barbae. Dermatol Ther. 2004;17:158–63.
4. Coley MK, Alexis AF. Dermatologic conditions in men of African ancestry. Expert Rev Dermatol. 2009;4:595.
5. British Association of Dermatologists. Pseudofoliculitis. Patient Information Leaflet; 2016.
6. Kauvar AN. Treatment of pseudofolliculitis with a pulsed infrared laser. Arch Dermatol. 2000;136:1343–6.
7. Grossman MC. Damage to hair follicles by normal-mode ruby laser pulses. J Am Acad Dermatol. 1996;35:889–94.
8. Sadighha A, Mohaghegh Zahed G. Meta-analysis of hair removal laser trials. Lasers Med Sci. 2009;24:21–5.
9. Hendrick C, Alster TS. Comparison of long-pulsed diode and long-pulsed alexandrite lasers for hair removal: a long-term clinical and histologic study. Dermatol Surg. 2001;27:622–6.
10. Schulze R, Meehan KJ, Lopez A, et al. Low-Fluence 1,064-nm laser hair reduction for pseudofolliculitis barbae in skin types IV, V, and VI. Dermatol Surg. 2009;35:98–107.
11. Smith EP, Winstanley D, Ross EV. Modified superlong pulse 810nm diode laser in the treatment of pseudofolliculitis barbae in skin types V and VI. Dermatol Surg. 2005;31:297–301.
12. Ross EV, Cooke LM, Overstreet KA, et al. Treatment of pseudofolliculitis barbae in very dark skin with a long pulse Nd:YAG laser. J Natl Med Assoc. 2002;94:888–93.
13. Alster TS, Bryan H, Williams CM. Long-pulsed Nd:YAG laser-assisted hair removal in pigmented skin- a clinical and histological evaluation. Arch Dermatol. 2001;137:885–9.
14. Alexis AF. Lasers and light-based therapies in ethnic skin: treatment options and recommendations for Fitzpatrick skin types V and VI. Br J Dermatol. 2013;169:91–7.
15. Leheta TM. Comparative evaluation of long pulse alexandrite laser and intense pulsed light systems for pseudofolliculitis barbae treatment with one year of follow up. Indian J Dermatol. 2009;54:364–8.
16. McGill DJ, Hutchison C, McKenzie E, et al. A randomised, split-face comparison of facial hair removal with the alexandrite laser and intense pulsed light system. Lasers Surg Med. 2007;39:767–72.
17. Bouzari N, Nouri K, Tabatabai H, et al. The role of number of treatments in laser-assisted hair removal using a 755nm alexandrite laser. J Drugs Dermatol. 2005;4:573–8.
18. Bouzari N, Tabatabi H, Abbasi Z, et al. Hair removal using an 800-nm diode laser: comparison at different treatment intervals of 5, 60 and 90 days. Int J Dermatol. 2005;44:30–53.
19. Lanigan SW. Incidence of side effects after laser hair removal. J Am Acad Dermatol. 2003;49:882–6.
20. Nanni CA, Alster TS. Laser assisted hair removal: side effects of Q-switched Nd:YAG, long-pulsed ruby, and alexandrite lasers. J Am Acad Dermatol. 1999;41:165–71.
21. Abdulmajeed A, Shapiro J, Rivers JK, et al. Paradoxical hypertrichosis after laser epilation. J Am Acad Dermatol. 2005;53:85–8.
22. Gauglitz GG, Korting HC, Pavicic T, et al. Hypertrophic scarring and keloids: pathomechanisms and current and emerging treatment strategies. Mol Med. 2011;17:113–25.
23. Alster TS, Tanzi EL. Hypertrophic scars and keloids. Am J Clin Dermatol. 2003;4:235–43.
24. British Association of Dermatologists. Keloids. Patient Information Leaflet; 2017.
25. Al-Attar A, Mess S, Thomassen JM, et al. Keloid pathogenesis and treatment. Plast Reconstr Surg. 2006;117:286–300.
26. Roseborough IE, Grevious MA, Lee RC. Prevention and treatment of excessive dermal scarring. J Natl Med Assoc. 2004;96:108–16.
27. Leventhal D, Furr M, Reiter D. Treatment of keloids and hypertrophic scars- a meta-analysis and review of the literature. Arch Facial Plast Surg. 2006;8:362–8.
28. Khatri KA, Mahoney DL, McCartney MJ. Laser scar revision: a review. J Cosmet Laser Ther. 2011;13:54–62.
29. Shokrollahi K. The laser test patch: principles and philosophy to maximise efficacy and reduce complications and scarring from laser treatments. Ann Plast Surg. 2016;77(4):373–5. https://doi.org/10.1097/SAP.0000000000000894.

Informed Consent for Laser Therapy in Scar Management

Youssof Oskrochi, David Bodansky, Kayvan Shokrollahi, and Adeyinka Molajo

1 Introduction

The aim of this chapter is to provide an overview of consent as relevant to laser therapy. This is especially relevant because lasers and laser treatment can be complex and difficult to explain, may require multiple sessions and have a distinct risk of complications that can be mitigated through good communication, safe practice and appropriate documentation.

2 Legal and Ethical Issues Relevant to Consent

Autonomy is the overriding principle of consent and is the absolute right of an adult with capacity to make informed decisions about their own care. Two conditions must be met for a decision to be regarded as autonomous; it must be free from external influence and made with the presence of mental capacity. The consenting physician must be satisfied that the decision has been made without duress; methods include speaking to only the patient face-to-face with a nurse or other healthcare professional as a chaperone, or asking their general practitioner or other involved healthcare personnel for their advice.

The legal principles of Mental capacity are presented in Table 1.

Y. Oskrochi
Royal Liverpool and Broadgreen University Hospitals NHS Trust, Liverpool, UK
e-mail: youssof.oskrochi@nhs.net

D. Bodansky
Department of Orthopaedic Surgery, Royal Liverpool Hospital, Liverpool, UK

K. Shokrollahi (✉)
Burns and Plastic Surgery Unit, Whiston Hospital, Liverpool, UK

A. Molajo
Mersey Regional Centre for Burns and Plastic Surgery, Whiston Hospital, Liverpool, UK

Table 1 Requirements for mental capacity

Mental capacity as defined in the Mental Capacity Act 2005
1. Understand the information relevant to the decision
2. Retain that information
3. Use or weigh that information as part of the process of making the decision, or
4. Communicate his decision

If informed consent cannot be achieved, the practitioner must act in the patient's best interests. An Independent Mental Capacity Advocate (IMCA) should be considered in certain circumstances such as where there are no friends, family or next of kin to contribute to decision-making. In Montgomery *v* Lanarkshire Health Board (UK Supreme Court 2015), the importance of discussing all the alternatives to the proposed treatment was highlighted.

3 Obtaining Consent in Laser Scar Management

Appropriate communication is fundamental in the transfer of that information, and problems in communication are the most often reported reason for patients making formal complaints. Communication should be targeted to patient level of understanding and avoiding technical terms. Asking the patient to explain what they know is a good starting point as this allows the physician to gauge not only their understanding but also their level of language that the patient is comfortable with. Treatment will be more successful if patients understand and can comply. Patients will also be better informed and treated more safely after test patching is undertaken.

Risks and Benefits: The most important aspect of the consent process is for the patient to be fully informed of the potential benefits and the risks associated with the planned procedure. The benefits should be discussed early in the consent process with care taken not to overemphasise the effect as this may unrealistically increase patient expectations and

K. Shokrollahi (ed.), *Laser Management of Scars*, https://doi.org/10.1007/978-3-030-52919-2_16

Table 2 The required topics that should be covered and documented in the Informed Consent Procedure

Topics that should be covered and documented in the Informed Consent Procedure
• The condition/disorder/disease that the patient is having/suffering from
• Necessity for further testing
• Natural course of the condition and possible complications
• Consequences of non-treatment
• Alternative treatment options available (Montgomery ruling)
• Potential risks and benefits of treatment options
• Duration and approximate cost of treatment
• Expected outcome
• Follow-up required

may lead to subjective unsatisfactory outcomes post-treatment. Similarly, the risks and complications should be plainly and honestly stated. Written material is encouraged, as is a consultation and window of opportunity ('cooling off period') for patients to consider information prior to commencing treatment. A Cochrane review on the use of decision aids made specific mention to their ability to improve patient knowledge and develop more realistic outcomes.

Documentation: Although taking informed consent culminates in a signature on a form, the documentation leading up to this signature must not be taken for granted. Meticulous and clear documentation of every stage of the consent process is paramount. Documentation with respect to consent should offer a clear and detailed summary of the discussions had, the parties present and the dates and location in which they took place. The content of this documentation should be able to provide evidence beyond doubt that the requirements of informed consent as set out in Table 2 were met.

4 Informed Consent in the Laser Treatment of Cutaneous Scarring

For any consent to be valid, it needs to be informed. Informed consent involves a frank and honest discussion of the potential risks and benefits of the suggested treatment with the patient. Here, we have provided guidance on the benefits and complications of laser scar management which should be discussed and documented in keeping with the principles outlined earlier in this chapter.

Benefits: The benefits of the proposed procedure need to be identified and documented, with special consideration given to the realistic expectation from the procedures. Patients need to be informed that they can expect an improvement in the visual appearance of the scar, but that there may not be total resolution.

Risks: The common side effects and complications of the procedure must be discussed; however, the rare but potentially serious complications must also be discussed if these may be of relevance to the patient.

Lack of Benefit: Patients should be warned that the procedure may not result in the benefit that they seek and this must be made clear. Realistic expectations should be discussed, and anonymised examples of previous typical outcomes should be shown to the patient. The discussion must be clearly documented both in the consent and medical notes. Test patching can feed into this.

Expected Post-Treatment Response: Post-treatment erythema, pain, petechiae/purpura and serous exudate and bleeding can all be the normal physiological responses to some laser treatments.

4.1 Burns and Blisters

Burns and blisters from non-ablative laser treatments can lead to scarring and dyspigmentation and test patching is strongly advised prior to treatments to maximise safety and patient expectations.

Prolonged Post-Operative Erythema: If the duration of erythema exceeds approximately a week with non-ablative resurfacing (<1% incidence) or 1 month with ablative resurfacing (23–33% incidence), it is termed prolonged post-operative erythema. Risk factors for its development include multiple laser passes or unintentional stacking. Prolonged post-operative erythema may remain for up to 3 months but should resolve without intervention, although topical anti-inflammatories may be useful. Er:YAG lasers often cause less post-operative erythema, likely due to the more superficial nature of treatment, when compared to CO_2 lasers.

Infection: Viral, bacterial and fungal infections may occur and usually present within the first 7 days post-operatively. Complications of infected laser sites include delayed wound healing, scarring and systemic infection. HSV infections are the most common (0.3–2% fractionated lasers, 2–7.4% unfractionated lasers) and often present as superficial erosions at the treatment site, rather than the classic herpetiform vesicles. The role of prophylactic antiviral medications is controversial; although prophylaxis has been widely recommended, some data does not support its use, citing similar HSV reactivation rates between previously exposed individuals given antivirals (6/86, 7%) and those exposed but not given antivirals (8/173, 4.6%).

Bacterial infection rates are extremely low (0.5–4.5%, 0.1% for fractionated), and the most common organisms responsible are *Staphylococcus aureus* and *Pseudomonas aeruginosa*, usually precipitated by excessive wound dressings and sealing. Proper identification, investigation including swabs and management with topical or systemic antibiotics are important in preventing further complications such as impetigo or systemic spread and secondary infection. Extra care should be taken in the immunosuppressed, and prophylactic antibiotics may be considered.

Fungal infections are rare but are usually caused by Candida species when they do occur. These usually manifest later than viral and bacterial infection, normally 7–14 days post-treatment and require antifungal management to prevent scarring.

Post-Inflammatory Hyperpigmentation: Often seen in patients with darker (Fitzpatrick III–VI) skin types or those with recent tanning, its occurrence after any laser procedure is possible with an estimated incidence of 1–37%. Procedures which involve ablative resurfacing are particularly prone to this phenomenon and patients should be warned that it is a common occurrence. Most often, hyperpigmentation is temporary and will often resolve within 3–4 months. Topical bleaching (hydroquinone) or peeling agents (retinoic acid, ascorbic acid, glycolic acid) may be used to hasten resolution, and patients should be advised to avoid sun-exposure to the affected areas and use copious amounts of sunscreen.

Hypopigmentation: As with hyperpigmentation, hypopigmentation can occur after any laser procedure although it is extremely uncommon. However, it is more common after intervention involving pigment-specific or melanin-targeting wavelengths. The extent of hypopigmentation in these cases is usually dose-dependent. In non-pigment targeting cases, hypopigmentation may have a delayed onset up to 1 year later.

Scarring Including Hypertrophic Scarring and Keloids: All laser treatments can cause scarring, but this is seen most frequently from ablative laser treatments. Of the non-ablative lasers, long-pulsed Nd:YAG laser using smaller spot sizes is a particular risk, as are all Q-switched lasers. Scarring is mitigated by test patching then treatment with parameters that are the same or very similar with small increments. Operator-dependant risk factors include lack of technical experience or training, use of new lasers, and lack of test patching whilst patient factors include concomitant local infection, history of keloids, skin type 4–6, previous local radiation exposure or surgery, previous herpes infection, a range of dermatological conditions and various medications including:

- Photosensitisers
- Immunosuppressants
- Retinoids

For ablative lasers, neck skin is particularly at risk of scarring due to the presence of fewer pilosebaceous units from which the healing process and re-epithelisation occurs.

Cicatricial Ectropion: A similarly rare but distressing complication often affects the eyelids and results in eversion of the inferior eyelid away from the eye with subsequent corneal exposure. Risk factors include previous surgery or excessive skin laxity around the eye and early ophthalmology involvement is required.

5 Consent Pitfalls

Shortfalls in the consent process are a leading cause of complaints and litigation claims. The consent process is designed to ensure patients are fully aware and understand the potential benefits and complications of their procedure. It is therefore not surprising that when patients do complain with respect to their treatment, deficiencies in the consent process have often contributed. Broadly these complaints with regard to consent appear to be divided into four categories:

Discussion of Complications: The most often cited reason for complaints, in one study 70% of surgical patients cited the lack of awareness of complications as a reason for complaints or clinical litigation claims.

Lack of Benefit: The second most common reason is that patients argue that they were not informed about the possibility that the intervention will result in any noticeable improvement and therefore underwent a procedure, with associated risk, for no gain.

Consent Procedure: Finally, a significant portion of complaints also centred around the process of obtaining consent, specifically patients feeling rushed or not being in the correct state of mind—especially if immediately before a painful or stressful procedure. Test patching as part of a cooling off period prior to treatment is good practice and will avoid such issues. A request-based method of consent is also a good way of ensuring understanding and documenting consent in patients' own words.

6 Conclusion

A well-informed patient will be aware of complications and have a good understanding of the realistic outcomes they can expect from treatment as well as what the alternatives are. Documentation of the informed consent procedure is very important, and clinical photography, test patching and written information are important contributors to a quality consent process for laser treatment.

Further Reading

Alster T, Zaulyanov L, Zaulyanov-Scanlon L. Laser scar revision: a review. Dermatol Surg. 2007;33(2):131–40.

Avram MM, Tope WD, Yu T, Szachowicz E, Nelson JS. Hypertrophic scarring of the neck following ablative fractional carbon dioxide laser resurfacing. Lasers Surg Med. 2009;41(3):185–8.

Bernstein LJ, Kauvar AN, Grossman MC, Geronemus RG. The short- and long-term side effects of carbon dioxide laser resurfacing. Dermatol Surg. 1997;23(7):519–25.

Bismark MM, Gogos AJ, McCombe D, Clark RB, Gruen RL, Studdert DM. Legal disputes over informed consent for cosmetic procedures: a descriptive study of negligence claims and complaints in Australia. J Plast Reconstr Aesthetic Surg. 2012;65(11):1506–12.

Consent: patients and doctors making decisions together. General Medical Council; 2008. ISBN: 978-0-901458-31-5.
Fife DJ, Fitzpatrick RE, Zachary CB. Complications of fractional CO2 laser resurfacing: four cases. Lasers Surg Med. 2009;41(3):179–84.
Fisher GH, Geronemus RG. Short-term side effects of fractional photothermolysis. Dermatol Surg. 2005;31(9 pt 2):1245–9; discussion 1249.
Gilbert S. Improving the outcome of facial resurfacing--prevention of herpes simplex virus type 1 reactivation. J Antimicrob Chemother. 2001;47(Suppl T1):29–34.
Gogos AJ, Clark RB, Bismark MM, Gruen RL, Studdert DM. When informed consent goes poorly: a descriptive study of medical negligence claims and patient complaints. Med J Aust. 2011;195(6):340–4.
Goodwin APL, Martin IC, Shotton K, Mason KM. On the face of it: a review of the organisational structures surrounding cosmetic surgery [Internet]. National Confidential Enquiry into Patient Outcome and Death; [cited 2015 Sep 22]. Available from www.ncepod.org.uk/2010report2/downloads/CS_report.pdf.
Gorney M. Scar: the trigger to the claim. Plast Reconstr Surg. 2006;117(3):1036–7.
Graber EM, Tanzi EL, Alster TS. Side effects and complications of fractional laser photothermolysis: experience with 961 treatments. Dermatol Surg. 2008;34(3):301–5; discussion 305–7.
Mamelak AJ, Goldberg LH, Marquez D, Hosler GA, Hinckley MR, Friedman PM. Eruptive keratoacanthomas on the legs after fractional photothermolysis: report of two cases. Dermatol Surg. 2009;35(3):513–8.
Nanni CA, Alster TS. Complications of cutaneous laser surgery. A review. Dermatol Surg. 1998;24(2):209–19.
Nanni CA, Alster TS. Complications of carbon dioxide laser resurfacing. An evaluation of 500 patients. Dermatol Surg. 1998;24(3):315–20.
Patel AJK, Morrison CM. Opportunities to reduce plastic surgery claims through an analysis of complaints data. J Plast Reconstr Aesthetic Surg. 2013;66(4):455–9.
Stacey D, Bennett CL, Barry MJ, Col NF, Eden KB, Holmes-Rovner M, et al. Decision aids for people facing health treatment or screening decisions. Cochrane Database Syst Rev. 2011;(10):CD001431.
Shokrollahi K, Ann R. Request for treatment: the evolution of consent. Coll Surg Eng. 2010;92(2):93–100. https://doi.org/10.1308/003588410X12628812458851.
Tierney EP, Hanke CW. Treatment of CO2 laser induced hypopigmentation with ablative fractionated laser resurfacing: case report and review of the literature. J Drugs Dermatol. 2010;9(11):1420–6.

Legal Cases

Montgomery *v* Lanarkshire Health Board, given by the UK Supreme Court on 11 March 2015.
Sidaway v. Board of Governors of the Bethlem Royal Hospital [1985] AC 871.
Chester v Afshar [2004] UKHL 41.

Complications Including Scarring Caused by Lasers

Kayvan Shokrollahi

No treatment or intervention is without risk. The only way to completely avoid any complication is never to treat. In certain circumstances, not treating can be the best option for a range of reasons beyond the scope of this chapter.

When lasers do offer potential improvements for patients, it is important to:

- Detail the risks and benefits to that patient in an understandable way.
- Ensure the risk: benefit ratio is proportionate.
- Ensure consent is undertaken properly (see the chapter on consent).
- Ensure that an appropriate history and medical examination is undertaken.
- Ensure that the mental health of the patient is taken into consideration.
- Ensure test patching is undertaken if/when appropriate (see chapter on test patching).

The potential complications or reactions from laser treatment depend on the laser and the treatment undertaken, but include the following:

Acute:

- Pain.
- Burns/blisters.
- Erythema.
- Sensitivity to ultraviolet and other radiation (heat).
- Temporary or permanent hair loss.
- Ocular injury.

Delayed/subacute:

- Scarring.
- Pigmentary change (hypopigmentation or hyperpigmentation).
- Temporary or permanent hair loss.
- Paradoxical hair growth.
- Infection.
- Bleeding.
- Erythema.
- Iatrogenic patterns on the skin from the laser.

Laser treatments are often undertaken in conjunction with other modalities and this fact should be taken into account when undertaking laser treatment.

Strategies to minimise the risks and dealing with the various side effects or complications of laser treatment include:

- Pain
  Ancillary cooling; ancillary oral analgesia; topical local anaesthesia; appropriate laser settings; distraction methods; good operator technique.
- Burns/blisters
  For non-ablative lasers, the best strategy is to undertake test patching and repeat test patching if significant increases are made to laser parameters before undertaking larger surface areas of treatment. In addition, ancillary cooling; appropriate laser settings.
- For ablative lasers, the thermal injury sustained is akin to a burn. An open wound and loss of contiguity of the skin are expected and part of the intended therapeutic strategy. It is therefore not a complication of ablative treatments to have an open wound similar to a burn.
- Erythema
  Non-ablative laser treatments usually cause a degree of immediate diffuse erythema which settles typically after a few hours. Treatments using short pulse durations at purpuric settings of the pulsed dye laser will leave more substantial erythema, often in the pattern of the laser spot, which can take some days to resolve. It is important to forewarn and also to acknowledge that men are typically not armed to mitigate this problem using make-up in the

K. Shokrollahi (✉)
Burns and Plastic Surgery Unit, Whiston Hospital, Liverpool, UK

K. Shokrollahi (ed.), *Laser Management of Scars*, https://doi.org/10.1007/978-3-030-52919-2_17

same way as female patients undertaking the same treatment.
Ablative or resurfacing treatment can result in prolonged periods of erythema.
It is again important to forewarn and also to acknowledge that men are typically not armed to mitigate this problem using make-up in the same way as female patients undertaking the same treatment.

- Sensitivity to ultraviolet and other radiation (heat)
  Avoidance of sun exposure is at the top of most pre-and post-laser instructions for patients. Patients may be uncomfortable, but may sustain significant pigmentary issues especially hyperpigmentation, if there has been significant pre-treatment sun exposure, or if they sustain sun exposure after treatment.
- Temporary or permanent hair loss
  Collateral damage to hair follicles can occur when lasers are being used in any hair-bearing area.
  It is important to ensure patients understand when they are likely to lose hair temporarily, or whether permanent hair loss or reduction might ensue when hair is not the target of therapeutic intervention.
- Ocular injury
  Appropriate eye protection must be utilised at all times.
  The two main types of ocular injury are retinal injury and corneal injury. Treatments around the eye may necessitate use of intraocular eye shields.
- Scarring
  Test patching will limit the potential for scarring and also assist with the choice of appropriate laser parameters to maximise therapeutic gains.
  CAUTION: There is substantial potential to cause extensive scarring in the process of treating lesser or minor scarring with lasers. Such scenarios include acne scars of the face and burn scars. It is better to undertake multiple or a series of test patches, than to cause complications.
- Pigmentary change (hypopigmentation or hyperpigmentation)
  Hypopigmentation can occur most frequently in patients with darker skin types, whilst hyperpigmentation is even more common in this patient group.
  Post-inflammatory hyperpigmentation (PIH) is very difficult to treat, resolves in an often-prolonged timeframe and causes significant consternation from patients.
  If after test patching there is signs of PIH, one should reconsider laser treatment as a suitable modality, or test patch again with a different strategy.
- Temporary or permanent hair loss
  Counsel patients so they are aware that most hair loss in areas of laser treatment is not permanent. In areas where it could be problematic, such as treatments in the hairline or eyebrows that appropriate precautions should be taken and consent obtained.
- Paradoxical hair growth
  Paradoxical hypertrichosis has been described. This is typically related to hair removal treatments.
- Infection
  Infection is only generally a risk from ablation and resurfacing treatments. Good skin hygiene prior to treatment and an appropriate aftercare regime should be sufficient. Prophylactic antibiotics are used by some, but this is controversial. Antivirals to limit the potential risk of reactivation of herpes virus, in particular those with a history of cold sores, are often prescribed.
- Bleeding
  Laser treatment using ablative lasers, which are surgical lasers, can cause acute or delayed bleeding.
  Non-ablative lasers can result in bleeding when they have been used to treat vascular lesions.
- Photosensitivity reactions
  Some medications and herbal remedies can cause photosensitivity and subsequent burns or blisters at otherwise safe laser settings, or despite appropriate test patching. A drug history is important [12], especially new drugs that have been started.
- Mental health
  It must be acknowledged at the outset that patients' mental health can be significantly impacted by scarring. There are many treatment factors that can impact patients that must be taken into consideration and discussed/explained with them, and possibly require a mental health professional's opinion and involvement if not already. These include:
    Expectations of the treatment and what can and cannot be achieved.
    Pain and other factors such as burning smells during the treatment.
    Pressure for repeated treatments with no end points.

1 Treatment of Scars Caused by Lasers

Whilst this book focusses on laser scar management, I would urge caution in relation to treating a scar caused by a laser with more laser treatment—especially the same laser.

There may be scope for using alternative laser strategies in some instances, but with clear goals and with test patching at the forefront of the strategy.

Further Reading

1. Shokrollahi K. The laser test patch: principles and philosophy to maximise efficacy and reduce complications and scarring from laser treatments. Ann Plast Surg. 2016;77(4):373–5. https://doi.org/10.1097/SAP.0000000000000894.

2. Fife DJ, Fitzpatrick RE, Zachary CB. Complications of fractional CO2 laser resurfacing: four cases. Lasers Surg Med. 2009;41:179–84.
3. Willey A, Anderson RR, Azpiazu JL, Bakus AD, Barlow RJ, Dover JS, Garden JM, Kilmer SL, Landa N, Manstein D, Ross EV, Sadick N, Tanghetti EA, Yaghmai D, Zelickson BD. Complications of laser dermatologic surgery. Lasers Surg Med. 2006;38(1):1–15.
4. AlNomair N, Nazarian R, Marmur E. Complications in lasers, lights, and radiofrequency devices. Facial Plast Surg. 2012;28(3):340–6.
5. Nanni CA, Alster TS. Complications of cutaneous laser surgery. A review. Dermatol Surg. 1998;24(2):209–19.
6. Metelitsa AI, Alster TS. Fractionated laser skin resurfacing treatment complications: a review. Dermatol Surg. 2010;36(3):299–306.
7. Zelickson Z, Schram S, Zelickson B. Complications in cosmetic laser surgery: a review of 494 Food and Drug Administration manufacturer and user facility device experience reports. Dermatol Surg. 2014;40(4):378–82.
8. Weisberg NK, Greenbaum SS. Pigmentary changes after alexandrite laser hair removal. Dermatol Surg. 2003;29(4):415–9.
9. Barkana Y, Belkin M. Laser eye injuries. Surv Ophthalmol. 2000;44(6):459–78.
10. Jalian HR, Jalian CA, Avram MM. Common causes of injury and legal action in laser surgery. JAMA Dermatol. 2013;149(2):188–93.
11. Chandrashekar BS, Shenoy C, Madura C. Complications of laser and light-based devices therapy in patients with skin of color. Indian J Dermatol Venereol Leprol. 2019;85:24–31.
12. Drucker AM, Rosen CF. Drug-induced photosensitivity: culprit drugs, management and prevention. Drug Saf. 2011;34(10):821–37. Review. PubMed PMID: 21879777. https://doi.org/10.2165/11592780-000000000-00000.

GPSR Compliance

The European Union's (EU) General Product Safety Regulation (GPSR) is a set of rules that requires consumer products to be safe and our obligations to ensure this.

If you have any concerns about our products, you can contact us on ProductSafety@springernature.com

In case Publisher is established outside the EU, the EU authorized representative is:

Springer Nature Customer Service Center GmbH
Europaplatz 3
69115 Heidelberg, Germany

Batch number: 10731524

Printed by Printforce, the Netherlands